Irina Spirina
Tat'qna Kowalenko
Elizaweta Fauzi

ASPECTS OF SOME PATHOGENETIC MECHANISMS OF SCHIZOPHRENIA

Irina Spirina
Tat'qna Kowalenko
Elizaweta Fauzi

ASPECTS OF SOME PATHOGENETIC MECHANISMS OF SCHIZOPHRENIA

CLINICAL-PSYCHOLOGICAL AND IMMUNOLOGICAL FEATURES

ScienciaScripts

Imprint

Any brand names and product names mentioned in this book are subject to trademark, brand or patent protection and are trademarks or registered trademarks of their respective holders. The use of brand names, product names, common names, trade names, product descriptions etc. even without a particular marking in this work is in no way to be construed to mean that such names may be regarded as unrestricted in respect of trademark and brand protection legislation and could thus be used by anyone.

Cover image: www.ingimage.com

This book is a translation from the original published under ISBN 978-620-4-20104-7.

Publisher:
Sciencia Scripts
is a trademark of
Dodo Books Indian Ocean Ltd., member of the OmniScriptum S.R.L Publishing group
str. A.Russo 15, of. 61, Chisinau-2068, Republic of Moldova Europe
Printed at: see last page
ISBN: 978-620-4-05110-9

MINISTRY OF EDUCATION OF UKRAINE

PRIVATE HIGHER EDUCATION INSTITUTION

"DNIPRO HUMANITARIAN UNIVERSITY"

SPIRINA I. D., KOVALENKO T.Y., FAUZI E. C.

ASPECTS OF SOME PATHOGENETIC MECHANISMS OF SCHIZOPHRENIA

(Clinical-psychological and immunological features)

Monograph

2021

CONTENTS

INTRODUCTION

Schizophrenia is one of the most important problems of modern psychiatry. One of the proofs of this can be a large number of scientific studies, which are conducted in all countries of the world in order to clarify its nosological boundaries, search for the causes and peculiarities of its appearance and development, develop new methods of treatment and social rehabilitation of patients. The diversity of classifications, interpretations of clinical symptomatology by different schools of psychiatry indicate that to date there is no unified view on the etiology, pathogenesis and clinic of schizophrenia. In the words of Lopes Ibor "...schizophrenia is enigmatic as a sphinx, it is a mystery...".

The leading method for diagnosing this disease to date is the clinical and psychopathological method [35, 36, 37, 53, 62]. The main attention of researchers was directed to the study of the clinical picture of psychosis. The fact of schizophrenia was considered only as a situation in which schizophrenic psychosis developed.

Numerous studies carried out by various authors to identify the "biochemical substrate" in schizophrenia indicate changes in many types of metabolism in this disease. However, attempts to detect the underlying metabolic defect to date have not yielded the desired result. Laboratory methods for diagnosing schizophrenia are lacking. A study of the literature devoted to the problem of biochemical diagnosis of schizophrenia shows that this problem remains poorly studied; the results of studies are scattered and insufficient in most cases.

All this is a stimulus to search for new biochemical tests, specific biochemical markers, which could be used to improve diagnosis and control the effectiveness of treatment of schizophrenia patients. The development and introduction into psychiatric practice of additional tests for diagnosis and prognosis of this disease enables specialists to reach a qualitatively new level of research and practical work.

Recently, a comprehensive biochemical approach has been used in the study of mental disorders. One of the promising methods is the detection of neurospecific antigens in the biological fluids of patients. The working hypothesis of our study was the assumption that only from the standpoint of a systematic approach it is possible to reveal regularities of clinical and immunological relations in various forms of schizophrenia in order to concretize a holistic view of their role in the pathogenesis of the disease. In turn, this will allow to allocate complexes of the interconnected clinical, immunological and psychological signs significant for diagnostics and the course of disease prediction, treatment efficiency increase and remission stabilization. It has been shown that the prevalence of schizophrenia, its clinical development and pathogenetic mechanisms are not determined by any one specific clinical, social, genetic or immunological factor, but are a consequence of their integral correlations.

Clinical-diagnostic and therapeutic significance of the obtained data consists, first of all, in the fact that on the basis of the results obtained specific differentiated complexes of clinical, immunological and social indexes, remission course are given, the realization of which allows to improve the quality of diagnosis and the effectiveness of rehabilitation measures.

SECTION 1.
LITERATURE REVIEW

The special medical and social significance of schizophrenia is explained by the fact that it is a problem of millions of patients with manifest forms of the pathological process, which affects mainly people of young and middle age, 0.85-1% of the world's population. Schizophrenia affects people of all social strata. Each year $14 per patient is spent on schizophrenia research ($300 for each cancer patient). This is a very "lopsided" "allocation of money", as schizophrenia costs society more than all oncology combined [27, 28].

The importance of the problem increases manifold if we take into account, as the data of psychiatric centers of the developed countries testify, that for 1 case of obvious schizophrenia there are approximately 3 latent, latent cases, and that special difficulties are connected with the absence of clear additional preclinical criteria capable of maximum objectification of its verification. Despite the existing achievements in the development of schizophrenia doctrine, the issues of etiopathogenesis, clinic, treatment and rehabilitation of patients with this progredient disease remain a topical area of psychiatry.

In different periods of the development of world psychiatry, the works of psychiatrists were dominated by biological and sociological concepts that considered the causes of schizophrenia, its course, recovery and outcome processes in two directions - biological and social.

However, there is another, opposite direction, characteristic mainly of psychiatry in Western countries, reflecting social concepts of schizophrenia. Many representatives of this direction connect the emergence, spread and development of the disease with socio-demographic, economic, cultural, family factors and "life stresses".

Studies concerning the study of "life events" in the occurrence of schizophrenia are important for the further development of psychosocial concepts of the disease. However, these studies are associated with great difficulties in defining "life stress", its assessment, methodological difficulties, etc.

Meyer (1951) held the view that schizophrenia is simply a form of "reaction" to stressful life events.

Most psychogenic theories assume that schizophrenia is caused by etiological factors" that either constitute stress, or decrease stress tolerance, or interact.

These results have also been confirmed by American studies in which newly admitted schizophrenic patients experienced significantly more significant life events during the six months preceding hospitalization than did controls. Evidence for the importance of life events preceding acute schizophrenic illness in its development is, for example, the repeated observation that the incidence of schizophrenia among emigrants varies inversely with the interval of time since emigration. Similar findings were obtained in an analysis of the results found in a survey of U.S. Army personnel hospitalized with a diagnosis of schizophrenia. The incidence was found to be significantly higher in the first months of service compared to the second year.

The relationship between critical life situations and schizophrenia has also been shown. In the life of large schizophrenic patients before their hospitalization, almost twice as many complicating situations (change of workplace, moving to another place of residence, childbirth, wedding, death, etc.) are found compared to the control group.

On   the basis of more than 140 observations, it has been shown that the judicial situation is often a contributing factor to the detection of ongoing schizophrenia. In this case, the first manifestations of the illness reflect either the situation as a whole or its separate sides [22, 32, 62].

It should be emphasized that, despite numerous studies in this field, the authors of the mentioned works were not able to make definitive conclusions about the role of environmental factors in the development of schizophrenia and their place in the pathogenesis of the disease. This is probably due to the great methodological difficulties in performing the research, as well as to the difficulties in interpreting the results obtained. The latter is further complicated by the fact that at present there are many works in which researchers do not find a significant influence of environmental factors on the development of schizophrenia.

So R.N. Nosk (1960), based on clinical observations, expresses doubt that schizophrenia is a disease of the poor and did not find dependence of frequency of occurrence of schizophrenic syndromes in people on their level of cultural development, that is, schizophrenia is revealed even in representatives of those tribes whose life is not influenced by modern civilization.

Gradually, the development of ideas about the causal relationship between environmental factors and schizophrenia has shifted toward the view that the differences observed reflect the course of schizophrenic illness rather than its origin.

According to the socio-ecological "drift hypothesis," schizophrenic patients who experience social difficulties as a result of their illness migrate to the slums of large cities and thus concentrate in squalid neighborhoods and accumulate among low social groups.

A more detailed study of first-time hospitalized patients shows that social deterioration often precedes the onset of illness. Those who are ill are not socially disadvantaged from birth. They suffer from moral and physical disabilities that impair their success in school, putting them at a disadvantage compared with others in achieving a working career.

Schizophrenia is not so much characteristic of the lower class as it contributes to the descent of the social ladder, due to the inability of patients to adapt to the demands of life.

Thus, despite the diversity of biological, genetic, and sociological studies, all questions concerning causality in the pathogenetic mechanism remain unresolved.

The interpretation of data from unilateral genetic studies is also not always clear-cut. Proponents of the hereditary theory of schizophrenia see these data as evidence for heredity theory, whereas proponents of psychodynamic concepts see evidence for the predominant role of the environment.

At the same time, much evidence suggests that environmental social factors may be partially responsible for the development of schizophrenia in genetically predisposed individuals [119].

It is theorized that the development of schizophrenia is determined by organic factors and that psychogenic factors may precipitate it. Primary symptoms, such as certain thought disorders, are thought to be of organic etiology, whereas secondary symptoms, such as certain types of delusions, are determined by psychiatric factors (188).

A comparison of the nature and importance of life events that precede the onset of schizophrenia and those that precede the onset of depression or suicide attempts suggests that the pathogenic effect of such events leads: to schizophrenic illness in some, to depression in others, and to a normal adaptation response in most. And so must be considered in relation to each individual's predisposition to illness.

The cause of schizophrenia must be viewed holistically, as the result of interdependent and interdependent factors that reinforce or potentiate each other, and may also weaken or even eliminate themselves.

C. Barley (1968) presented a schematic representation of the etiology of schizophrenia, involving the interaction of various physiological, psychological and social stressors against the background of the organism's genetic predisposition to the disease, which leads to specific brain dysfunction and the development of the disease.

G. Gross, G. Huber, and Scgutler (1971), supporting the view of situationally independent ontogeny in most schizophrenic patients, found in 23% of the 557 patients studied a clear relationship in time between mental or somatic factors and the primary manifestation and remanifestation of psychosis. In 39 of 175 patients with schizophrenia with affective onset, the authors also found psychoses in their families, indicating a possible role of genetic factors in the disease.

H. Heimann (1975) summarizing questions about the possible role of environmental environmental, social, intrafamilial factors on the basis of his own research and data from other authors, suggests a model in which a known genetically determined predisposition influences the specificity of schizophrenic syndromes and, together with a range of non-specific mental stresses, forms a single, complementary system.

We propose a model of schizophrenia that would combine modern psychosocial and biochemical-physiological research findings. Possible points of contact between these mechanisms, in the author's opinion, could be biogenic amines that are intensely released under mental stress and their quantitative and possibly qualitative fluctuations lead to the development of schizophrenia-like symptoms [143].

M. Strahilevits (1974) considers manifestations of the clinical picture of schizophrenia as a result of interaction of stressful environmental factors with genetic predisposition to pathology of biological processes in the patient's organism.

Reciprocal intertwining of genetic and environmental factors in schizophrenia S. W. Matthysse, (1976) see a hereditary "basis-deficit" of the biochemical homeostasis system causing clinical manifestations of schizophrenia" as a result of various stressful situations (early negative environmental influences, cultural and socioeconomic deficiencies, mental overload, somatic diseases).

On the basis of genetic data, Huber (1976) concludes that brain metabolism disorders, or rather defects in enzyme metabolism, which cause special sensitivity of the brain to environmental influences, are inherited and determine the appearance of schizophrenia. As the author notes, various somatic and mental stresses, causing a "shift" of the hereditary predisposition beyond the threshold zone, provokes schizophrenic psychosis.

There is also a concept of schizophrenia in which proponents have evidence for an important role of immunological mechanisms in the genesis of the disease. Some studies emphasize the relationship between changes in immunoglobulin concentrations and stressors. Thus, Hendric, Parashevas, Varramis (1972) associate an increase in plasma IgA concentration with the occurrence of anxiety. Similar data were obtained in a study of patients with polyarthritis, which allowed the relationship between serum immunoglobulin levels and the number of life events that can be considered as stressful. It was concluded that stress can increase serum immunoglobulin A levels.

Given the discrepancy in the results obtained by different authors when studying immunoglobulins in schizophrenia, it is probably worth remembering that immunoglobulin levels are a stable and genetically fixed intrafamilial trait; therefore, fluctuations in this parameter in the same patient at different periods of the disease rather than the average values of immunoglobulin concentration in different patient groups should probably be given more importance. Other studies also indicate that stress can lead to hypofunction of the immune system and increase the permeability of the blood-brain barrier [123].

Using immunofluorescence method, autoantibodies (immunoglobulin G) that bind to antibodies of the septal region of the brain of schizophrenia patients

were detected. The obtained data allowed the authors to refer schizophrenia to autoimmune diseases [158].

Other authors do not support an autoimmune model of schizophrenia, but point to the need for further immunological research into the etiopathogenesis of the disease.

If autoimmune processes in relation to brain tissue are associated with schizophrenia, are they related to genetic and environmental influences.

The role of hereditary factors in the development of immunological shifts in schizophrenia is evidenced by the frequency of detection of humoral anti-brain complement-binding autoantibodies in patients and their closest relatives [97].

Hereditary causation of immunological disorders in schizophrenia is established according to the detection of antibodies to DNA in the blood sera of first-degree relatives of probands [76]. The findings also mean that genetic factors are involved in determining individual differences in the level of antithymocytic activity of serum in patients with schizophrenia as assessed by indirect fluorescence [97].

However, as it turned out, the development of immunological processes may be determined not only genetically, but also by the influence of various non-specific environmental factors.

Based on the above, we can conclude that the influence of the environment on the development of schizophrenia may be mediated through the activation of autoimmune processes, changes in immunoglobulin content and permeability of the blood-brain barrier under stress.

The emergence of data on the involvement of neuroendocrine factors in the regulation of the human immune system functioning was the starting point for the development of studies, currently denoted as "psychoimmunology" or "psychoneuroimmunology", in which the relationship and interdependence in the functioning of the immune, endocrine and nervous systems are studied.

It has also been suggested that an immunological approach to the study of schizophrenia runs through the "crossroads" of research into the role of the environment, including the possible influence of a hypothetical schizophrenia virus, and the importance of hereditary predisposition   for the development of the disease [149].

The data presented and the opinions of various authors on the considered issues of schizophrenia etiopathogenesis show that neuroautoimmune processes arising in the organism of schizophrenia patients, both in connection with hereditary predisposition and in response to non-specific influences from the external social environment, may be one of the possible points of contact between genetic and environmental, social and biological factors in the pathogenesis of schizophrenia.

The peculiarities of interaction between social and biological in the "organism-environment" system are described as follows: "the integrity of an organism, the composition and interaction of its components, thus, act as a result of not only the external environment, fixed in heredity, but also the internal activity of the organism itself, its ability to adaptive changeability" [16].

Based on the dialectical interpenetration of biological and social in man himself, the division of the causes of disease into external and internal is erroneous and, in fact, makes no sense. All diseases, including hereditary ones, were eventually formed, consolidated and transmitted from generation to generation during the active interaction of man as an organism and a personality, with his nature and social environment [53, 107].

The founders of Russian psychiatry outlined a correct understanding of the relationship between social and biological factors in mental disorders. Thus, as early as V.P. Serbsky (1900) pointed to the "bad sides of civilization" as the cause of growth of mental diseases, considering heredity, trauma, poisoning and various acute and chronic somatic diseases as their direct causes.

It is known that one of the independent directions of studying the biological bases of schizophrenia is the study of neuroautoimmune processes, which is evidenced by clinical and immunological correlations established by different authors, as well as experimentally discovered membranotropic and neurotropic properties of blood sera of patients whose activity is considered in connection with the presence of   anti-brain autoantibodies [2, 37, 43, 52, 76, 83, 103, 138, 145, 156, 157, 158, 159, 160, 182, 190]. However, previous studies have not provided an unequivocal answer to the question of whether the immunological shifts detected in schizophrenia belong to protective reactions of the organism or are immunological processes involved in the development of the disease.

The discrepancies concern not so much the general ideas about the importance of neuroautoimmunity in schizophrenia in general, but also individual immunological indicators and the clinical and immunological correlations established by different authors with the clinical form, severity of course, acuteness of condition, efficiency of therapy, stability of remissions and their prognosis.

No relationship has been found between   the frequency of detection of complement-binding anti-brain autoantibodies in the sera of patients and the type of course of schizophrenia, but a higher level of these autoantibodies is observed in the intermittent course compared with the continuous-gestational course, In contrast, complement-binding autoantibodies have been found to be relatively more frequent in the continuous and seizure-progredient course and very rarely in the intermittent course, as in healthy controls [43, 75, 96].

A possible explanation for such discrepancies may be not only peculiarities of immunological research methods, but also differences in the criteria for dividing schizophrenia into separate clinical forms and conducting research in heterogeneous samples of patients who happened to be in the same hospital at some period and therefore this contingent was not sufficiently repreventive.

In addition, when describing certain clinical and immunological correlations, other clinical data about the patient and the course of the disease, as well as those environmental factors that may have influenced certain immunological parameters, were not always taken into account simultaneously. Thus, it is now established that the neuroautoimmune shifts detected in schizophrenia can be both genetically and caused or activated by various psychiatric and somatic aggressors [76, 96, 97, 164].

Consequently, the immunological shifts detected in schizophrenic patients reflect changes in various interrelated parts of the immune system that are closely related to other body systems and the environment, i.e. they represent a "crossroads" or one of the points of contact between these internal and external systems. Therefore, analyzing the results of previous clinical and immunological studies of schizophrenia, a critical attitude to the attempts to   directly compare immunological shifts with clinical features of the disease, which "are far from providing direct evidence of the existence of direct links between the corresponding processes, for they are mediated by many biological systems" is established [157].

To take into account simultaneously correlations of various but interrelated clinical, genetic, immunological and social factors in pathogenesis and course of schizophrenia is possible only with the system approach to a subject of research" that, as underlined psychiatrists, developing methodological questions of psychiatry, allows to avoid one-sidedness of investigation, to reveal general, connected into a single whole mechanism of development of disease, its internal laws and their interrelation with environment [111, 118, 157, 173].

The correlation of social and biological in the pathogenesis of mental disorders should be considered from the recognition of the "unity of etiology and pathogenesis" [152].

Pathogenesis in its essence is a biological phenomenon, but this does not mean ignoring the influence of social factors on its mechanisms. Thus, pathogenesis in the system of medical cognition is considered as a sociobiological mechanism of disease, which is determined simultaneously by natural and social factors, which allows us to highlight the structure of "formed systems" and reflect the restructuring of functions and the state of the human body [3].

As it turned out, many processes that outwardly look "purely" biological ultimately depend on social factors. This is also true for disorders of immunological reactivity, which play an important role in the pathogenesis of schizophrenia.

The immune system, designed to maintain the constancy of the antigenic composition of the organism, protection from alien genetic information and thereby ensure the constancy of the internal environment, is an extremely sensitive mechanism, quickly responding to relatively weak but evolutionarily unexpected factors (O.V. Baroyan, 1978). Therefore, the isolation of an internal factor, immunological reactivity, from the causal interaction by no means means means ignoring other elements, including environmental factors [73].

Thus, the position on the unity and dialectical interaction of social and biological factors in the etiopathogenesis of disease is one of the fundamental methodological and scientific methodological principles that help to bring clarity to the direction of theoretical research and practical work in modern psychiatry.

At the same time, the role of social and biological factors is different in different mental illnesses and at different stages of their development, and their components are nonindetrimental. Therefore, psychiatry faces the task of concretely deciphering this formula, taking into account the nosological clinical form of the disease [90, 111, 152].

It is known that if a disease is a combined process of an adverse environmental impact and the organism's response to it, then the task of the researcher is to address both the analysis of environmental factors and the study of the organism's reactivity [155].

It is possible to reveal these features of interaction of internal and external, biological and social in etiopathogenesis of schizophrenia only on the basis of scientifically grounded system approach which main attribute is understanding of integrity of human vital activity, his health and illness.

In the theory of pathology the systems approach involves not only a holistic consideration of the social and biological in the human body system, but also the interaction of systems - the human body and its surrounding social environment".

Only systemic medical cognition allows one to approach the pathological process, its occurrence, course, reversal or other outcome in the unity of its biological and social aspects, in the unity of the individual, the organism and the environment, which is the best means of avoiding errors in scientific research.

The systemic approach excludes the opposition, "splitting" of the integrity of human health and disease into social and biological, or reduction of one to the other, which contradicts the dialectical understanding of the relationship between these two forms of motion of matter, reflecting the system of interaction and mutual mediation in a complete body and in its relationship with the environment.

The task of systems research also determines a fundamentally new cognitive situation, which is characteristic of modern science. If in the pre-systemic studies it was a description of the object, the systemic studies are aimed at revealing the mechanism of "life" of the object, highlighting previously unknown functional and structural formations, which often fundamentally changes our understanding of the process [51].

The integrative trends presented in the systems movement are a natural response to the deepening specialization of medicine to obtain or maintain a holistic picture of human pathology.

The importance of revealing the internal relationships between symptoms, signs, which "in mathematical language is equivalent to assumptions about the presence of a certain hidden structure of relationships of symptoms", was emphasized, in particular, by a well-known expert on the application of mathematical methods in biology and medicine [20].

The theory of systems in its application to tasks of psychosomatic researches demands obligatory consideration of all set of the phenomena of human life.

The reconstruction using mathematical methods and description of such systems is one of the ways, besides experimental and mathematical, of system modeling of the pathological process.

Consequently, the urgent needs of psychiatry development, on the basis of modern deeper and more complex, multilevel and multidimensional scientific knowledge correspond to a systematic approach to the object of research - the pathological process and its life activity.

Therefore, successful solutions to many of psychiatry's problems can be accomplished through a synthesis of clinical psychiatry and the allied sciences of the patient, both body and person - biological and social psychiatry.

In the pathogenesis of schizophrenia, the major role of various metabolic disorders (protein, lipid, carbohydrate, catecholamines, and endorphins), autoimmune processes, glial cell areactive and diffuse neuronal death in the large hemisphere cortex, and neurodynamic processes   was noted [10, 22].

Disruption of lipid peroxidation plays a leading role in the mechanisms of autoimmune disorders in schizophrenia [46].

Although fundamental ideas about the possibility of immunological mechanisms involvement in the onset of mental illnesses were expressed as early as 1903 by V. Seletsky, systematic studies of this issue were initiated in 1937 by Leman-Facius. He found antibodies to brain tissues in the serum and cerebrospinal fluid of schizophrenic patients, which became a serious guide to the development of immunobiological concepts of schizophrenia.

An important role of complex immunological shifts **in the pathogenesis of schizophrenia has been concluded** [159, 160]. The presence of allergies to neurohormones, including adrenaline, in schizophrenic patients may indicate a direct link between this phenomenon and the development of general neuroallergy, since according to the existing concept, allergic processes in tissues proceed with the release of adrenaline and nadrenaline [13, 112].

It is known that CNS, in particular brain, as a source of autoantigens is a rather peculiar organ. The brain tissues are isolated from contact with immunogenic formations of the organism. They belong to those tissues, morphological and functional differentiation of which comes rather late. These circumstances aggravate the so-called foreign properties of mature brain antigens. In pathological processes in the CNS accompanied by destructive phenomena, together with other products of cell destruction the proteins of nervous tissue

will be excreted into the bloodstream. The presence of nerve tissue proteins in the serum has been shown [81, 104].

The onset of the schizophrenic process, both in its primary case and in its relapse, is associated with the appearance of brain antigens and neutrophils sensitized by them in the blood serum, which can be considered as a stage of neurosensitization of the organism due to the developed destructive processes in the brain tissues [168].

In these cases, an urgent appropriate reaction - the appearance of anti-brain antibodies - signifies the onset of a stage or phase of protective-adaptive reactions of the immunocompetent system aimed at restoring the damaged homeostasis. The appearance of serum antibodies in the immunized organism is preceded by the emergence of a population of lymphoid tissue that carries cellular antibodies. Such lymphocytes are the carriers of tissue immunity [80, 104]. Humoral antibodies represent the final stage in the development of immunogenesis processes, at this time great importance is given to the cellular mechanisms of immunopathological process that precede the formation of humoral antibodies [168].

During aggravation of the process, destruction of brain tissue occurs, causing the appearance of brain antigens, which have an excitatory effect on CNS, both directly and indirectly through histamine [160]. Histamine realizes the action of antigen on tissues and cells of the histiocytic reticuloendothelial system. Presumably, the accumulation of biogenic amines, primarily histamine, leads to an increase in the permeability of the blood-brain barrier and promotes the release of brain antigens into the cerebrospinal fluid and bloodstream. In this case there is a direct effect of humoral antigens on basophilic leukocytes, reticulocytes and others with subsequent production of anti-brain antibodies.

At present, an essential role of hereditary factors in the development of schizophrenia can be considered proven, and naturally, the question arises about a possible connection between immunopathological shifts in schizophrenia and hereditary factors in this disease, especially since the intensive development of immunogenetics has proved the genetic dependence of immunoglobulin synthesis [77, 105].

The results of the studies undoubtedly indicate a significant role of genetic mechanisms in the formation of humoral antibodies against antigens to brain tissue. Two mechanisms are the real ones:

it is possible that genetic factors predisposing to schizophrenia determine the appearance of a special clone of lymphoid cells sensitive to a minimal amount of neural tissue protein of the brain responsible for the production of overt anti-brain antibodies released into the bloodstream as a consequence of physiological dissimilation processes;

hereditary increase in permeability of membranes of nerve elements of the brain in the patient with schizophrenia should lead to regular and sufficiently intensive release of proteins beyond the boundaries of cell barriers of the organ into the bloodstream. Their next contact with lymphoid elements will lead to the formation of antibodies.

In this case various stress factors, to which the cells of the normal organism will respond with less intensive, fast reaction, the nervous elements of the patient in the consequence of the caused increased membrane permeability will constantly serve as a source of brain antigens to support the immunopathological processes. It is known that the existence of insignificant stress situations, with the mechanisms described above, can give this process a chronic character [105].

Immunological abnormalities in schizophrenia are associated with both cellular and serum protithelial antibodies [104].

In schizophrenia, the level and functional ability of T-lymphocytes is reduced more than that of B-lymphocytes [78].

The study of leukocyte cultures obtained from schizophrenia patients found that immunological reactions of delayed-type hypersensitivity regarding brain antigens develop in the organism of patients, which are accompanied by an increase in the number of circulating immune lymphocytes in the bloodstream [95, 168].

Among lymphocytes of patients with schizophrenia a separate part of cells is characterized by signs of sensitization to antigens of nervous tissue. Sensitization is manifested in the ability of lymphocytes to cause lysis of nervous tissue elements in vitro. This proves the fact of cytotoxic action of lymphocytes of patients with schizophrenia [161, 104].

The study of peripheral blood lymphocytes in patients with schizophrenia revealed the existence of cell subpopulations with different signs of activation. An increase in the percentage of lymphocytes with atypical morphology, an increase in the number of lymphocytes with elevated RNA synthesis intensity and chromatin activation, and the content of adhesive lymphocytes was sharply elevated [147].

In the organism of schizophrenia patients, the number of subpopulations of adherent lymphocytes, i.e., lymphocytes that are in the activated state, exceeds the number of adherent cells in peripheral blood of healthy donors by 2.4-fold [107, 147].

The following types of immunograms have been identified:

Type 1, brain antigens only,

Type 2 - only antimouse circulating autoantibodies;

Type 3 - only indicators of cellular sensitization to the brain;

Type 4 - both brain antigens and circulating brain antibodies;

Type 5 is both circulating antibodies and cellular sensitization to the brain;

Type 6 - both brain antigens and indicators of cellular sensitization to the brain.

Mental deterioration was observed more frequently among patients with immunogram types 4 and 6 (45% and 37.5%), when brain antigens and indicators of cellular sensitization to the brain were detected simultaneously. These immunogram variants reflect not only the process activation, but also the specific immunopathological reactivity of the organism [114].

Delayed cell reactivity turns out to be the first stage of all immunological reactions, which is usually followed by antibody formation. Thus, the immunological process can be imagined in the following way: under antigenic influence on the organism, populations of immunologically active cells appear among a large number of nonimmune lymphocytes, which can react directly with antigens at the first stage and give rise to antibody-forming cells at the stages that come later.

The acuteness of the course of the schizophrenic process, the degree of its progredient, the rate of development of clinical manifestations can be related to the individual properties of the reactivity of the organism and, in particular, to the rate, intensity and sequence of the appearance of neurosensitization and neuroimmune response [167].

The degree to which immunological parameters deviate from the norm allows for a deeper assessment of the nature of psychopathological manifestations in schizophrenia [145].

Impaired immunobiological reactivity contributes to the progressive course of schizophrenia and aggravates its clinical manifestations [78].

In the early stages of the schizophrenic process, autoimmunization of the organism by brain antigens is accompanied by pronounced allergic components, which considerably increase the acuteness of the process [159].

The type of schizophrenia treatment is determined by the rate of development of neuroallergic reactions, their speed, and mobilization [168].

The presence of anti-brain antibodies simultaneously in the serum and cerebrospinal fluid of a patient with schizophrenia characterizes the severity of the disease [95, 166].

Changes in the immunological reactivity of the organism were found in schizophrenia patients not only during exacerbation of the process, but also in remission [114].

Activation of the dopaminergic system or blocking of other systems (serotonergic, cholinergic, GABAergic) lead to an increase in the intensity of immunological reactions and improvement in the mental state of schizophrenic patients. On the contrary, blocked defaminergic system and activation of the above three systems, negatively affect the size of immune reactions, cause deterioration of the mental state of patients [10].

Many studies suggest that a variety of antibody types (anti-brain, pro-tymphocyte, pro-stimphocyte, etc.) may be formed in schizophrenia. Non-specific and generalized proteins appear in the blood and cerebrospinal fluid and autoantibodies are found in the blood, cerebrospinal fluid, and brain tissue. Atypical P-lymphocytes have been detected in the blood of schizophrenia patients, and the well-known idea that this phenomenon is related to neuroleptic use is rejected [117].

Antibodies are known to have the following three main functions in terms of their properties:
Have protective properties
To be mere "witnesses"
Have aggressive properties [8].

The assignment of protithelial antibodies detected in schizophrenia to one of these groups may determine their role in the mechanism of disease development.

Evidence suggests that cellular antibodies from lymphocytes of patients with schizophrenia are capable of inducing damage effects in brain tissue culture cells [104].

The study of autoimmune shifts in the blood in paranoid schizophrenia shows that the dynamics of antibodies and antigens in the blood are characterized by their cyclic appearance and disappearance. In a prolonged study it is possible to identify up to 2-3 cycles of immunization of the organism with brain antigens [166].

A clear dependence of the frequency of the appearance of anti-brain antibodies with an increase in the psychopathological manifestations of the disease has been revealed [105].

In schizophrenia, the white matter proteins of the brain are most frequently, but not exclusively, and as it was not uncommon to combine with similar hyperreactivity to the gray matter of the cerebral cortex, and sometimes to the gray matter of the subcortex as well [159].

In patients with schizophrenia, a higher sensitivity of leukocytes to antigens obtained from the gray matter of the frontal and parietal parts of the brain of a deceased schizophrenic patient was found than in controls (healthy and neurotic patients). The authors reported the release of immunologically active RNA by these parts of the brain of the deceased [117].

A number of studies on the role of immune factors in the pathogenesis of schizophrenia have obtained data on an increase in the number of B-lymphocytes in peripheral blood due to mature cell forms. Along with an increase in the total number of B-lymphocytes, the number of cells synthesizing immunoglobulin, mainly of class G, significantly increases [151].

However, there are various conflicting data in the literature. It is proved that in primary schizophrenia patients only Ig G levels are higher than normal, in chronicity of the process - all three classes of Ig (A, M, G) [2].

Having studied the levels of Ig G, A and M in the plasma and cerebrospinal fluid of chronically ill patients, a greater concentration of Ig was found in them compared to controls (healthy individuals and neurologically ill patients) [117, 121].

Neuroimmune processes affect not only brain neurons but also neuroglia [168].

Enteral administration of blood serum of schizophrenia patients and Ig G isolated from it to rats leads to polymorphic changes in organelles of cytoplasm of neural glial and endothelial cells, synapses of membrane structures [161].

Ig G sera   from patients with schizophrenia have the ability to induce distinct changes in the ultrastructure of neurons and glial cells. The nature of ultrastructural abnormalities when injecting Ig G isolated from blood serum of dogs immunized with brain or myelin basic protein is different from those when injecting Ig G serum of schizophrenia patients. Leading the way is damage to myelin membranes [34].

Elevated Ig G levels in patients with schizophrenia may be seen as a reflection of the underlying process, or perhaps as a reaction to an exacerbation of the disease. High levels of Ig M are a component of the pattern of hereditary predisposition to schizophrenia. The serum fraction of patients with schizophrenia that has Ig M is significantly more pronounced than the corresponding fraction of healthy individuals, depolarizes and inactivates the neuronal membrane [107].

An increase in B-lymphocyte counts from initial levels during treatment is an unfavourable prognostic sign and clinically corresponds to a worsening condition (51).

It is known that, under normal conditions, the amount of immunoglobulins in serum is small, but significantly increases with prolonged stimulation of the immune apparatus [80, 81, 104].

As revealed by biochemical studies, the biologically active factor of the blood serum of schizophrenia patients was associated with the β-globulin fraction of proteins. In this region, schizophrenia patients appeared to have a pre-precipitation arc of a double-humped character. The first peak of this arc corresponded to β1-globulins and the second to β2-globulins. The fraction corresponding to the first peak was consistently present in all sera studied, while the other component was formed only in some of them. The detection of a labile β1-globulin component in the serum of schizophrenic patients suggests that this phenomenon is associated with immunological rearrangements in schizophrenic patients [105].

A   comparative immunochemical analysis revealed a difference in the levels of neurospecific β2-globulin in the cerebrospinal fluid of healthy and mentally ill patients. An increase in this protein in the cerebrospinal fluid is observed in patients with increased symptomatology in the paranoid form of schizophrenia, hallucinatory delusional and delusional syndromes. A decrease in neurospecific β2-globulin is observed with a decrease in symptoms [25].

In the initial stage of schizophrenia, it was found through immunoelectrophoretic studies that some serum   globulin fractions increased quite frequently [69].

In the initial stage, β2-globulins usually increase, which is seen as a response of the immunocompetent system.

Globulins were found to increase in 54% of patients examined, α1 fractions increasing from 6 to 10 g% in 28%, α2 fractions increasing from 10.5 to 15 g% and sometimes higher in 45%, and gamma globulins increasing from 19 to 25 g%, exceptionally higher in 29% [69].

In patients with an increase in globulin fractions of serum, a tendency to reach full remission was noted [69,114].

These observations suggest a possible prognostic value of the type and degree of immunoglobulin changes in schizophrenic patients.

During remission, after the first psychotic episode, there is a tendency for normalization of changes in the immunoelectrophoregram. Chronification of the schizophrenic process leads to an increase in α1-globulins. However, after a prolonged course of the disease (more than 6 years), these shifts flatten out and approach the norm [69, 145].

Antibodies that are constantly circulating in the blood of schizophrenic patients have a clear neurotropic effect, and as such can predetermine a variety of structural and functional abnormalities in the brains of these patients [34, 117].

Sensitization of lymphocytes to nervous tissue antigens has been established, which is manifested by spontaneous "blast"-transformation of lymphocytes of schizophrenia patients and their ability to cause damaging effects in brain tissue culture cells [29]. The latter circumstance (lysis of nerve elements) is particularly important because it indicates that antibodies against brain tissue not only have a protective function or indicate the presence of brain antigens in schizophrenia, but also prove to be "aggressive," capable of damaging healthy brain tissue [27, 28, 103].

Blood serum of schizophrenia patients has the revealed neurocytotoxic properties. Neurotropic action of serum corresponds to neurosensitization of T-lymphocytes on the background of decrease of their functional activity. Complement-binding antibodies are much less compared with cytotoxic ones which may indicate their different biological role. Hyperimmunoglobulinemia, which was detected in a significant number of patients (40%), was associated with complement-binding and, to a lesser extent, with cytotoxic anti-brain antibodies[161].

The biological significance of cytotoxic and complement-binding antibodies is unequal; it is possible to foresee that antibodies that produce a neurotropic effect are close in their characteristics to the type of antibodies that cause the reaction of neuroglia damage and other changes in the nerve tissue culture [165, 160]. Complement-binding antibodies that appeared against the background of the development of neurological symptoms and do not disappear in recovery can be referred to antibodies-witnesses [125].

The association between the clinical features of the disease and the presence of complement-binding antibodies indicates their possible pathogenetic role in the development of schizophrenia, which worsens the course of the pathological process [163].

The neurotropic effect of serum from schizophrenia patients may be due to the action of not only antibodies to brain antigens, but also antibodies to DNA [95].

Data on the revealed structural abnormalities in the brains of embryos from mothers with large schizophrenia and information on the association of perinatal brain pathology with neuroimmune conflict suggest that one of the causes of morphological changes in the brains of schizophrenia patients may be neurosensitization, and the main damaging factor is anti-brain antibodies [117].

It was shown that serum antibodies against brain tissue proteins, when introduced into experimental animals, can significantly change neurophysiological indicators of brain functions by fixation on the surface of cellular elements [105]. These data cannot be the final proof of the active role of immunological disorders in the pathogenesis of the disease, but they indicate a rather biological activity of the pro-tissue antibodies.

Remissions in patients with the paranoid form of schizophrenia with the presence of antibodies to the brain in blood serum are unstable. Antibodies in the blood of patients are indicators of an ongoing pathological process, which is associated with prolonged auto-sensitization of the organism by the products of brain tissue destruction [166].

When examining different types of schizophrenic remissions, the overall rate of detection of specific immunological shifts reaches 60%.
Remissions in schizophrenia are accompanied in some cases by incomplete extinction of pathological process, reduction of its activity.

The established relationship between the frequency of exacerbations of the disease and the results of previous immunological studies confirms this assumption and points to the active involvement of the immunopathological component in the development of exacerbations in schizophrenia [114]. In 1996, American scientists reported an increased concentration of the neurospecific protein N-CAM in the cerebrospinal fluid of schizophrenia patients [161].

Neuronal cell-cell adhesion protein (N-CAM) is involved in cell-cell interactions during synaptogenesis, morphogenesis and plasticity of the nervous system. Disruption of synaptic rearrangement and neuronal plasticity may be associated with the pathogenesis of some neuropsychiatric diseases, including schizophrenia. Impaired cellular function of the brain may alter the concentration of N-CAM protein in the cerebrospinal fluid.

A significant increase in N-CAM-immunoreactive proteins, primarily a band with a molecular weight of 120 kDa, in the cerebrospinal fluid of an inpatient with bipolar type 1 mental disorder and relapsing unipolar major depression has been reported.

No significant effect of drug treatment on N-CAM concentration was found. Pathological development of the CNS or brain damage later in life may cause impairment in the expression of N-CAM. The cerebrospinal fluid has relatively high concentrations of N-CAM protein, with the most prominent component N-CAM-120. Changes in synaptic rearrangement and neuronal plasticity may be related to the pathogenesis of schizophrenia [120, 121]. There was no correlation in the content of N-CAM in the cerebrospinal fluid depending on age and sex.

An increase in N-CAM content may serve as an indicator of increasing synaptogenesis. The formed brain can respond to damage by increasing synaptogenesis and synaptic reorganization.

N-CAM expression increases during these events. The increase in N-CAM in the cerebrospinal fluid of patients with schizophrenia may be associated with cellular rearrangements or possible degeneration of some cellular components of certain brain regions.

A review of the literature indicates a lack of unified views on the pathogenesis of the disease in its approach to its biochemical and immunopathological bases. The existing ambiguity and disagreement of ideas about the genesis of schizophrenia are due not only to the presence of many united pathochemical mechanisms, but also to diagnostic difficulties. At the current stage of development of the schizophrenia doctrine, the applied orientation of research to clarify its biology and pathoimmunochemistry, and the search for new additional diagnostic tests, the objectivity and validity of which will promptly decipher the pathogenesis of the schizophrenic process, are important. At the same time, diagnostic tests may not be firmly linked to the primary specific pathogenetic ring of schizophrenia. The "marker" may be a qualitative mapping of its pathochemical mechanisms (including secondary ones). It is important that the diagnostic complex and its constituent indices be strictly specific for a given disease and reliably distinguish it from psychoses similar in clinical symptomatology.

SECTION 2.

MATERIALS AND RESEARCH METHODS

2.1 Patient selection criteria

Selection of patients was carried out on the basis of Communal institution "Dnepropetrovsk clinical psychiatric hospital" of Dnepropetrovsk regional council. Criteria of selection were the following: female sex, age from 18 to 55 years, all patients were observed in inpatient conditions and gave their written consent to participate in the study. A total of 130 patients were selected for observation. Only women were included in the study, thus we achieved, firstly, homogeneity in the groups, secondly, female schizophrenia is more relevant, as it is considered more dangerous and unfavorable both for the patient and her offspring, and thirdly, initially no differences were observed in the immunological composition of the blood serum of male and female schizophrenia patients.

We selected women with paranoid and simple (neurosis- and psychopath-like) forms of schizophrenia, as these are currently the most common and, therefore, the most interesting to study in view of their pathomorphosis at the present stage. The control group included women with psychopathies and reactive psychoses.

The study group included patients with clinically confirmed diagnosis. Diagnosis was based on the synthesis of Kraepelin-Bleuler criteria, which corresponds to the principles of ICD-10 classification construction.

At the moment of examination all patients were in a state of aggravation of psychotic manifestations. Besides productive symptomatology, in a number of patients negative disorders were observed in varying degrees of severity in the clinic of the disease. More often they were shown in the form of emotional impoverishment, autism, reduction of energy potential, emotional inadequacy, loss of communicability.

Schizophrenia duration was 1-5 years in 20% (23 patients), 5-10 years in 25% (31 patients), over 10 years in 15% (30 patients). The control group accounted for 35% (46 patients) of all the studies.

All patients were examined using clinical and follow-up, clinical and psychological, and immunological methods. If as a result of research there were doubts in classification of the form, type of the course of disease, the patient was excluded from the group of the examined patients. Patients with somatic, endocrine and gross organic pathology were also excluded.

As a result, the described sample consisted of patients with clearly defined features of the disease and its course.

2.2 Clinical method

The diagnosis of the paranoid form is based on the phenomenology of content-related thinking disorders in combination with perceptual disorders. The clinical picture is characterized by relatively stable paranoid delusions, usually accompanied by auditory hallucinations, and other perceptual disorders. Syndromologically, the paranoid form, along with characteristic negative symptoms, is represented by paranoid, hallucinatory-paranoid, affective-paranoid (depressive-paranoid, expansive-paranoid) variants. Kandinsky-Clerambaut syndrome, whose components are included in R Schneider's list of first-rank symptoms, was at the forefront in terms of relative specificity among these syndromes. Elements of rudimentary psychotic symptomatology were often present during the manifestation stage of the pathological process. These manifestations were combined with formal thought disorders, most often in the form of autistic, paralogical, symbolic or magical thinking. The basis of diagnostics of the simple form of schizophrenia was detection of the following signs:

1) A distinct change in premorbid personality manifested by loss of drives and interests, inactivity, aimless behaviour, self-absorption and social autism;

2) Gradual emergence and deepening of "negative" symptoms - apathy, impoverished speech, hypoactivity, emotional stiffness, passivity and lack of initiative, poverty of non-verbal communication;

3) A marked decline in social, academic or occupational productivity.

Given the significant diversity in the course of schizophrenic disorders, the type of course of the disease was specified, and the results are reflected in Table 2.1:

Table 2.1

Distribution by type of course of schizophrenia

Type of flow	Total	1 gr.	2 gr.	3 gr.	4g.
Continuous rapid to moderate gradient	34	8	10	16	-
Seizure-progressive	43	15	14	14	-
Continuous low-grade	7	-	-	-	7

Continuous schizophrenia was characterized by remission-free dynamics, broad coverage of all registers characteristic of schizophrenia productive and negative disorders. The remissions are short "facade", medicated.

Seizure-progressive schizophrenia was characterized by seizures with affective components, a buildup of the defect from seizure to seizure, and remissions of varying duration with residual encapsulated symptoms.

The maloprogressive type of course was characterized by stable neurosis-like or psychopath-like symptoms, absence of delirium and hallucinations, absence of remissions, and unexpressed defectiveness.

The features of the initial period were investigated in the whole group. The average duration of disorders was 4.6±2.4 months. Among syndromes of the initial period there were neurosis-like, appearing in the form of neurasthenic and agripnic states, obsessive-phobic symptomatology, psychopathoid syndromes. Negative symptomatology was noted, the basis of which were phenomena of regression (reduction of energy potential) or regression of behavior to earlier ontogenetic stages of development (juvenileism, infantilism).

Pseudoorganic personality changes were manifested by "stupidity", lack of attention, uncorrigible mood swings, which were not determined by the environmental situation, and affective disorders in the initial period in the form of hypomania, apathetic subdepressions, apathetic subdepressions, and stale depressions with psychosomatic disorders.

In a small number of patients, the initial period was marked by erased psychotic episodes, whose fragmentation and lack of expansion made it impossible to speak of a manifestation period. These were episodes of delusional mood, supervised fixations, or brief episodes of non-targeted agitation during puberty. In one patient, a condition typologically similar to reactive-neurotic and following immediately after a psychotraumatic situation was observed.

Hallucinatory delusional symptomatology was noted in the form of a combination of delusions of persecution, attitudes and verbal hallucinosis. Kandinsky-Clerambaut syndrome was diagnosed with a combination of motor, ideational and sensory automatisms with delusions of exposure. The paranoid syndrome was represented by delusions of persecution, attitude.

Distribution by leading syndromes at the time of the study of the studied group of patients with schizophrenia in Table 2.2:

Table 2.2

Distribution by leading syndrome

Syndrome	Relative number	Abs. number, %
paranoid	26	22
hallucinatory-paranoid	56	47
paranoid affective	9	8
psychopath	4	3
neurosis-like	5	4

The distribution of patients with schizophrenia according to the age of illness is shown in Table 2.3:

Table 2.3

Distribution of patients with schizophrenia according to the age of illness

Age of illness	Absolute number	Percentage, %
1 month - 5 years	23	18
over 5 - 10 years inclusive.	31	24
over 10 years	30	23
control group	46	35
Total	130	100

It was the duration of the disease that formed the basis of the distribution of schizophrenia patients according to the level and severity of neurospecific protein responses.

Among symptoms, the first-rank symptoms according to C. Schneider are singled out due to their relative specificity for diagnosing schizophrenia.

Sperrungi, sounding of own thoughts, symptom of open thoughts, auditory antagonistic hallucinations, commenting auditory hallucinations were determined more often (Table 2.4).

Table 2.4

Distribution by first-rank symptoms

Symptoms	1 g, %	2 g, %	3 g, %	4 g, %
sperrung	33	62	85	16
somatic hallucinations	21	25	29	80
sounding of one's own thoughts	90	74	83	-
Auditory mutually exclusive and contradictory hallucinations	84	90	96	-
commenting hallucinations	90	85	77	-
mind control	98	89	84	-
the effects on the inducements	53	46	24	-
behavioural impact	73	86	57	-
effects on the senses	75	83	68	-
delusional fancy	88	76	43	-
symptom of an open mind	97	87	70	-

Only the leading first-rank symptoms are noted in the table.

Among the negative symptoms, mild changes in the form of emotional exhaustion and reduction of energy potential were diagnosed more often. The average duration of exacerbations ranged from 5 days to 7 months.

The quality of remissions was assessed by Sereisky:

- remission "A" was defined as remission without residual symptomatology.

"B" - remission with residual neurosis-like and psychopath-like symptoms, unexpressed negative disorders.

"C" - remission with residual productive symptomatology, "encapsulating delirium" syndrome, negative symptomatology.

"D" - change in the severity of psychopathological disorders of the psychotic period.

"O" - no change in the psychosis clinic within one year.

The distribution according to the quality of remission of the studied group of patients with schizophrenia is shown in Table 2.5.

Table 2.5

Distribution by quality of remission of the studied group of patients

Quality of remission	Absolute numbers	% of people with schizophrenia
«А»	18	21
«В»	44	52
«С»	5	6
«Д»	-	-
«О»	17	21
Total	84	

During exacerbation and during the first remission, patients received a variety of therapies and no measures of labor and social rehabilitation were taken. Therapy with psychotropic drugs was received by 70% of patients, of whom only one drug was received by 7% of patients, two drugs, including neuroleptic drugs and antidepressants were received by 43% of patients. More than two drugs from the group of neuroleptics were received by 30% of patients with schizophrenia. Therapy with psychotropic drugs in combination with insulincomatose therapy was received by 30% of patients.

In 51% of schizophrenic patients it was possible to describe defect syndromes.

In the structure of the defect there were distinguished: 1) psychopath-like type of defect; 2) apathetic-abulic type of defect; 3) mixed type of defect.

Other peculiarities of the clinic and disease dynamics of schizophrenia patients under study are given in the following chapters.

2.3 Psychological examination

Depending on the objectives of the study, we used three methods of experimental-psychological research:

1. Eisenk Personality Questionnaire.
2. The "incomplete sentences" technique.
3. The "nonexistent animal" technique.

Eisenk's test

EPI- Eysenck Personally Inventory - Eysenck Personality Inventory. Published in 1963, it consists of 48 questions for diagnosing extra- and introversion and neuroticism, as well as of 9 questions constituting the "lie scale", according to which a tendency to present oneself in a better light is determined. The test is designed to determine baseline personality dimensions. In this study, it determines the peculiarities of response and adaptation of the organism's psyche during the development of a disease, i.e. pathopsychological phenomena.

The questionnaire measures such mental properties as neuropsychic lability, level of extra- or introversion. Secondarily, we can deduce the presence of personality traits such as emotional stability and attribution of temperaments to classical types - choleric, sanguine, phlegmatic, melancholic. The questionnaire shows the relationship between these types of temperament and the results of the factor-analytical description of personality.

The technique contains 4 scales: extraversion-introversion, neuroticism and sincerity scale. The listed scales measure such features: extraversion is manifested in friendly, active, optimistic and confident communication; introverts are characterized by uncommunicative, passive, secretive communication. The average score on this scale is 12. Scores above 12 indicate extraversion, and scores below 12 indicate a tendency toward introverted behavior.

An individual with high neuroticism is characterized by hypersensitive reactions, tension, anxiety, dissatisfaction with oneself and the world around, and rigidity. An individual with a low level of neuroticism is calm, balanced, and at ease with communication. The average score on this scale is 8 to 16. Scores above 16 indicate a high degree of anxiety and mental instability.

The sincerity scale shows the degree of sincerity of the examinee, his/her attitude towards the survey. If the number of points exceeds 10, it is possible to speak about insincerity of the examinee.

The distribution according to the above parameters and the average values of the indicators in the studied groups are shown in Table 2.7:

Table 2.7

Average indicators of Eisenk's test in the studied groups

Average score	1 gr.	2 gr.	3 gr.	4g.	Counter.gr.
extra-introversion	8	6	3	7	15
neuroticism	30	27	29	18	15
sincerity	5	4	3	4	6

Thus, the dynamics of increasing level of introvertedness is traced according to the increase in the age of paranoid schizophrenia, while the level of anxiety remains the same. The degree of severity of these parameters was lower in group 4. The control group displays slightly less neuroticism and more extroverted behavior. A more detailed analysis can be found in the following chapters.

Incomplete sentences are used as a stimulus in order to identify feelings, attitudes, motives and needs in various significant areas of life. The test has a quantitative (positive or negative characteristic of the attitude system in scores) and qualitative (content analysis) assessment system.

The method includes 60 incomplete sentences that can be divided into 15 groups, which characterize the patient's system of relations to the family, to his/her own personality, to representatives of his/her own and the opposite sex, to superiors and employees.

Some sentence groups have to do with a person's fears and fears, their sense of guilt, their assessment of their past, present and future, their relationship with their parents and friends, their awareness of their own life goals.

For each group of sentences, a characteristic is derived that defines this system of relations as positive (+3, +2, +1), negative (-1, -2, -3) or neutral (0).

The distribution according to the above parameters and the average values of the indicators in the studied groups are shown in Table 2.8:

Table 2.8

Average values of the main scales of the "Unfinished sentences"

methodology in the studied groups

Basic scales	1 gr.	2 gr.	3 gr.	4g.	Counter. gr.
Attitude	0,3	-1,4	-2,2	1,1	2,1
Attitudes towards family	1,1	-1,3	-3	0,6	0,5
Attitude towards the past	0,3	-1,3	-2,2	0	1,7
Attitude towards the future	2,4	0,8	-1,9	1,6	2,4
Fears	-3	-3	-3	1	0,3
Guilt.	1,2	-1,7	-2,1	1,6	2

Thus, as the duration of paranoid schizophrenia increases, the tendency toward a decline in self-esteem (paraphrenic syndrome excluded), an increase in guilt, a worsening of attitudes toward the family, the past and the future, with persistent fears and apprehension   is traceable.

A more detailed description is in the next chapter.

The "Nonexistent Animal" method

Drawing a nonexistent animal is a projective technique for personality research proposed by M. Z. Drukarevich. It uses application of an indefinite stimulus, (to draw a nonexistent animal and call it by a nonexistent name) to diagnose personality traits of the subject. Indirectly determines the development of creative potential as well. The system of evaluation is not standardized, this study identified the most frequent features of drawings within, each group at the level of tendencies.

The research method is built on the theory of psychomotor connectivity. The study of motor skills (in particular, motor skills of the dominant hand that draws - fixed in the form of a graphic trace of movement, a drawing) is used to register the state of the psyche. According to I.M. Sechenov, any representation that occurs in the psyche, any tendency connected with this representation, ends with movement (literally: "Any thought ends with movement"). If actual movement for whatever reason does not take place, then a certain tension of energy is accumulated in the corresponding muscle groups, which is necessary to carry out the corresponding movement (per representation-thought). For example, imaginings and thought-imaginings that induce fear stimulate the tension in the leg muscle groups and in the arm muscles that would prove necessary in the case of a fear response by fleeing or defending with the arms - to strike, to shield. The tendency of movement has a direction in spaciousness: removing, approaching, bending, straightening, rising, falling.

When performing a drawing, the sheet of paper represents a model of space and, in addition to the state of the muscles, captures the attitude to space, that is, the tendency that emerges. Space, in turn, is connected with emotionally colored experiences and a time period: corresponding to reality, the past and the future. It is also related to the effectiveness or ideological and mental work plan of the psyche.

Besides general regularities of psychomotor connection and attitude to space, theoretical norms of operating symbols and symbolic geometrical elements and figures are used when interpreting test material. By its nature, this test belongs to the number of projective.

We chose to study the anxiety and aggressiveness levels as the main parameters of interest. The degree of expression of these parameters was taken in conditional units from 1 to 6. The results are shown in Table 2.9.

Table 2.9

Mean values of the main scales of the "Nonexistent animal" methodology in the study groups

Scales	1 gr.	2 gr.	3gr.	4g.	Counter.gr.
level of anxiety	6	5	5	3	3
level of aggressiveness	3	5	6	2	3

Detailed analysis in the next chapter.

2.4 Immunological method

All patients with a history of cerebral trauma or any organic brain lesions were excluded from the examination.

Blood from the patients was taken a few days after admission to the hospital, in the morning, on an empty stomach, centrifuged at 300 rpm. For 3 minutes. To determine autoantibodies the obtained sera were taken. To obtain the fraction of membrane and cytoskeleton neurospecific proteins, the brain of a healthy man who died as a result of a traffic accident was used (morgue of the Mechnikov Regional Clinical Hospital).

Membrane fraction preparation was prepared according to the following scheme: 1g of brain tissue was homogenized in 10 ml of buffer A (0.025 M Tris-NSL, with 7, 4, 2 m EDTA, 5 m soybean trypsin inhibitor, 0.1 m phenylmethylsulfonyl fluoride). The homogenate was centrifuged at 60,000g for 45 min. The supernatant was discarded and the precipitate was resuspended in buffer A and centrifuged again under the same conditions. The precipitate after centrifugation was resuspended in 2 ml of buffer A (0.025 M Tris-NSL, with 7, 4, 2 m EDTA, 5 m soybean trypsin inhibitor, 2% Triton X - 100 or 1% DCHL sodium dodecyl sulfate) and centrifuged at 60 000g for one hour. The supernatant thus obtained was used as a preparation of the membrane fraction. Immunoblotting method was used to determine the reaction of neurospecific antigens with serum antibodies.

Modern methods of one- and two-dimensional electrophoresis in gel systems, which contain detergents, allow efficient separation of hundreds of biopolymers, and solid-phase immunoassay and radioimmune assays show 10 g of substance (antigen) in one ml of solution. At that time the possibilities of analytical study of the nature and biological activity of individual molecules, distributed by electrophoresis, were limited, as the biopolymers localized in gel pores were not mechanically accessible, or chemically suitable for many types of subsequent analyses. Antigens that are located in the gel pores are not attainable for homologous antibodies, since the size of the latter is larger than the pore diameter of the matrix.

In 1979, a new technique was developed that allowed the separated molecules of the electrophoretic matrix to be pulled out, transferred and immobilized on the surface of the solid phase in the same order in which they were in the gel. As a result, a reflection (replica) of the electrophoregram, preserving the state achieved during electrophoresis, is obtained on the solid phase. The molecules that are studied are located in the gel thickness, and after the transfer is completed, they are concentrated on the surface of the solid phase and become available for subsequent analyses, the sensitivity of which is increased. During the transfer of biopolymers, it is possible to renaturate the molecules, which allows their nature, antigenicity, and biological activity to be analyzed. In determining the polypeptide composition of brain antigens, with which autoantibodies reacted with patients' serum, a dilution of 1:250 was taken.

Transfer time depends on gel thickness, porosity, and macromolecule size. At transfer from 12.5%-polyacrylamide gel of 1.5 mm thickness to membrane during one hour not less than 90% of proteins with molecular mass up to 90,000 are transferred. We chose to study the number and strength of reactions as the main parameters of interest, expressing these parameters in conditional units of 1 to 10.

The results of average indicators in each study group are shown in Table 2.10.

Average number and strength of immunological reactions on immunoelectrophoregrams

	1 gr.	2 gr.	3g.	4g.	Counter. gr.
Number of reactions	3,37	6.37	8,48	0,94	-
The power of immune responses	2,38	3,45	4,4	0,99	-

Thus, there is a clear pattern in the increase in the number and intensity of immunological reactions with increasing age of paranoid schizophrenia, and in the minimal presence of these indicators in simple low-progressive (neuro- and psychopath-like) form of schizophrenia. In the control group, this response is completely absent. A detailed discussion of the results of the examination in the following chapters.

SECTION 3.

CLINICAL-PSYCHOLOGICAL AND IMMUNOLOGICAL CHARACTERISTICS OF THE GROUPS IDENTIFIED

Depending on the severity of immunological reactions 5 groups were identified among the examined patients:

- group with no immunological response,
- group with a low-intensity response,
- a group that has a medium-intensity response,
- a group with a high intensity response,
- group of patients with the most pronounced reaction on immunoelectrophoregram.

Analysis of clinical examination results showed, as expected, that the group without antigens for neurospecific proteins in sera was composed of patients from the control group, i.e., individuals without schizophrenia whose diagnoses were other nosological units.

The remaining groups consisted of patients with schizophrenia. The main difference between the groups was the duration of the disease. In the group of 5-10 years old we identified a subgroup characterized by low intensity of immunological reaction, clinically it was represented by a simple form of schizophrenia - neurozo- and psychopath-like variant, with low-predictive type of course. All other patients had paranoid form and moderate-progressive type of course.

The groups of patients were combined as follows:

1. Patients with the paranoid form of schizophrenia with moderate progredient type of course, with duration of disease up to 5 years inclusive, having immunological reaction of blood serum on neurospecific proteins of medium intensity - 23 patients;

2. Patients with the paranoid form of schizophrenia with moderate-progressive type of course, with duration of disease over 5 to 10 years inclusive, having immunological reaction of blood serum on neurospecific proteins of high intensity - 24 patients;

3. Patients with the paranoid form of schizophrenia with moderate progredient type of course, with duration of disease more than 10 years, having maximal expressed immunological reaction of blood serum on neurospecific proteins - 30 patients;

4. Patients with the simple form of schizophrenia (neurozo- and psychopath-like variant), 5-10 years old, low-predictive type of course, low intensity of immunological reaction of blood serum to neurospecific proteins - 7 patients;

5. Control group - patients with psychopathies, reactive psychosis, no reaction of blood serum to neurospecific proteins - 46 patients.

3.1 Clinical and psychological characteristics of the identified groups

3.1.1 Clinical and psychological characteristics of group 1

All patients referred to the first group (23 patients) suffered from paranoid form of schizophrenia, the first exacerbation occurred relatively recently - from 1 to 5 years inclusive. The course of disease in the whole group was of moderate progredence, therefore only in - paranoid, including Kandinsky-Clerambaut syndrome; in 22% (5 cases) - paranoid syndrome, in 13% (3 cases) - depressive-paranoid syndrome.

In 35% (8 patients) the disease had a continuous, remission-free course; in 60% of patients there was an attack-progressive type of course. In 5% (1 case), the type of course was not established due to the short duration of the disease.

Progressive schizophrenia was observed after the age of 25, although there was an earlier (juvenile) manifestation. The disease developed slowly and gradually. Relatively acute onset was relatively rare - it was more characteristic of the continuous progenerative course of schizophrenia.

The initial stage of the disease was defined by individual obsessions, hypochondria, unstable, episodic or more systematized delusions (relationships, jealousy, etc.). Psychopath-like disorders were not uncommon during this period. Already at this time, personality changes noticed by others appeared: withdrawal, rigidity, loss of subtlety of affective reactions, emotional flattening. The range of interests gradually restricted, patients became distrustful, reserved, and sometimes gloomy. At times brief episodes of anxiety, restlessness with fragmentary ideas of attitude, persecution were noted. Further, usually after some years, delirium of persecution, physical influence, phenomena of mental automatism (Kandinsky-Clerumbo syndrome) appeared.

The clinical picture of the hallucinatory-paranoid syndrome characteristic of the manifest stage of the disease varied. In some cases, hallucinatory disorders prevailed (hallucinatory variant), and in others, systematized delirium of physical affect (delirium of Kandinsky-Clerumbo syndrome).

Hallucinatory variant of progressive schizophrenia. The first signs of developing hallucinosis: verbal illusions combined with delusional interpretation (self-referral) of others' speech. Then came elementary hallucinations, followed by verbal hallucinations, more often in the form of a hallucinatory monologue (the same voice talking about or addressing the patient, giving advice, scolding, ordering) or dialogue (several voices). Often the voices are multiple.

Pseudo-hallucinations and phenomena of mental automatism rather quickly increased. Development of Kandinsky-Clerambaud syndrome was gradual, or accompanied by aggravation of the condition with the appearance of fear, anxiety, agitation, confusion, elements of acute delirium, against which there was a feeling of openness (the patient's thoughts were known to others) and separate ideational automatisms. Later pseudo-hallucinations (mental voices, investing thoughts, etc.) prevailed. In addition, visual pseudohallucinations (evoked, made visual images), and senestopathic automatisms (evoked sensations in the body, internal organs) were not uncommon. The leading place was still occupied by verbal pseudohallucinosis. Delirium during this period was hallucinatory - its facet is closely connected with the content of voices (idem of influence, persecution, love delirium, etc.).

The emergence and development of Kandinsky-Clerambaugh syndrome was accompanied by a significant progression of changes - a distinct emotional defect, loss of social connections, increasing thinking disorders, discontinuity of speech. The course with more rapid change of stages, small systematization of delirium and rapid development of deep personality changes was observed at comparatively early onset of the disease (adolescence).

Delusional variant of progressive schizophrenia. Delusional disorders dominated throughout the disease from the moment of manifestation. In this case the disease developed gradually, debuting mostly in middle age. In more favorable cases for many years (sometimes decades) the clinical picture of the disease is limited by systematized delirium (of jealousy, reformation, invention, persecution, chicanery) without hallucinations and phenomena of mental automatism, i.e. all symptoms of sluggish paranoid schizophrenia described above. However, unlike the latter, periodic short-term exacerbations of the condition with the appearance of maliciously intense affect, elementary auditory and olfactory hallucinations, rudimentary, fragmentary automatisms (symptom of openness, senestopathic automatisms) are noted. The less favorable course of typical paranoid schizophrenia is not characterized by transient exacerbations, but by the transition of the paranoid syndrome to the paranoid syndrome. This may occur gradually by enlarging the delirium, by changing its facet, or after a short period of exacerbation.

Hallucinatory-paranoid syndrome. The clinical picture was characterized by delusions of exposure, sometimes having the character of physical, hypnotic, cosmic influence. Sensation of transfer of thoughts at a distance, influence by hypnosis, or invisible stations, transmitters, etc. was noted by patients. There were feelings of inserting or interrupting thoughts, events of past lives were unwittingly "unfolded". Specific disorders of thinking were characteristic, internal speech went out of control "someone speaks with his speech apparatus", internal conversations with others were conducted similar to "conversation with the mind" or "soul";

Hallucinatory syndrome: it was characterized by the predominance of verbal hallucinosis in the clinical picture, including "voices" of commentary, imperative, threatening nature. There were antagonistic, mutually exclusive hallucinations on a background of confusion, bewilderment, sense of fear. These patients were characterized by some isolation, they did not disclose their experiences. Under the influence of "voices" they performed absurd actions. There were pseudo-hallucinations in the form of "sounding thoughts", "echoes" and thoughts.

Part of the patients in this group had a state of "personality regression". This condition was characterized by the presence of deficit disorders along with residual productive symptomatology. Mental activity of these patients was characterized by monotony, some simplicity. Disturbances of associative processes were marked. Delusions and hallucinatory inclusions were unstable and stereotypical in their content.

The clinical features of this group are illustrated by the following example: Patient K., born in 1988. She is an only child in the family. Heredity was not burdened with mental diseases. Her early development had no peculiarities. Started school at age 7. Successfully completed 9 grades of secondary school. Entered into vocational school. Learned a profession - plasterer-painter. Worked on a specialty. She is sociable by nature, but touchy. Had many friends. Believes that she fell ill after she suffered a strong emotional shock - she caught her friend with another woman. That night she heard male "voices" inside her head scolding her and ordering her to "take off her clothes and shoes and run around at night. According to her mother, she changed her behaviour dramatically from February 2019. Stopped going out to work, was tense, anxious, suspicious, did ridiculous things, threw away clothes, refused to take food, listened to something, or suddenly froze staring at one point. She changed in relation to her mother, kicked her out of the house, claiming that she was jinxed. On June 16 suddenly, in the middle of the night, she pounced on her mother, trying to strangle her, even grabbed the night, but then burst into tears and told her mother that "the voices were forcing her to death," because they explained that it was not her mother but the girl her sweetheart was seeing. Sobbing asked her mother's forgiveness, she explained what had happened as an imposition, the evil eye, she did not know where the voices were coming from. For a week after the incident she was quiet, thoughtful, retiring, talking to herself, eating selectively, explaining that she had been given "such an instruction. On June 30, she again became tense, restless, cried and laughed for no reason, stripped naked, sometimes swore profanely, tried to run away from home half-dressed, got into a fight with her mother, although previously such behavior was not peculiar to the patient. On September 2, 2019, she was brought to the psychiatric ward by her relatives.

Mental status: Consciousness is not impaired. Accessible to contact. At the beginning of the conversation, she was excited, rushing around the room, striking herself, swearing cynically. She gradually calmed down, but looked anxious and confused. She tried to tell about her worries, explaining that "inside there was homesickness, anxiety, and voices from nowhere. At home the "voices" said that I would be killed and my mother was bad, she should be killed too. And now the "voices" are different - they talk about God, "I will accept faith together with them". I believed that it was sent from above. She noted that now she "knows everything ahead, she can foretell the future - I close my eyes and see everything that has happened and will happen in my memory; the events of the present and past are scrolled before my eyes". During the conversation, she often kept silent and closed her eyes. She denied misbehavior at home. Criticism of her experiences was absent. Intelligence corresponded to the education received.

Somatic condition: Average height, asthenic build, moderate nutrition. Skin is pale, moist. Heart tones were rhythmic. BP 125/75 mm Hg. Pulse 86 beats per minute. The lungs had vesicular breath sounds. No abnormalities of the internal organs were detected.

Neurological condition: Cranial nerves without pathology, tendon reflexes lively, identical in symmetrical parts of the body. Coordination disorders, pathological reflexes were not detected.

Diagnosis: Schizophrenia, paranoid form, hallucinatory-paranoid syndrome, seizure-progressive type of course.

When analyzing the first rank symptoms, it was found that the patients of this group were characterized by the presence of:

- auditory antagonistic hallucinations in 61% (14 patients);

- commentative auditory hallucinations in 65% (15 patients);

- spherung in 32% (7 patients);

-impact on inducements - in 37% (13 patients);

- sounding of own thoughts was noted by 56% (13 patients) of this group;

- the symptom of open-mindedness is characteristic of 50% (11 patients) of this group.

Among the negative symptoms, mild changes in the form of emotional impoverishment, mild thought disorders prevailed in 21% (5 patients), changes in the form of predominant regression were noted in 7% (2 patients).

Results of psychological research of group 1

Processing results of the Eysenck test (EPI), show low values on the scale "introversion-extroversion" (3-8 - "introvert", "potential introvert"). These values in this group reflect difficulties in interpersonal contacts resulting in withdrawnness, noncommunicativeness, striving for activities unrelated to communication, and anxiety reactions when forced contacts are made regardless of the subject's will.

With a decrease in social spontaneity, there is a tendency to prefer a narrow circle of close people to a wide range of contracts, and there are also difficulties in establishing new social contacts and anxiety reactions in case of social friction.

Moderately elevated values on the neuroticism scale (12-18) reflect the presence of internal tension, anxiety, potential for rapid change of mood, and lack of adaptation to surrounding conditions. In addition, such values on the neuroticism scale may correspond to feelings of anxiety, preoccupation, and depressive reactions.

The analysis of repeating elements in the drawing of the "nonexistent animal" (preference for a left-handed orientation of the object) allows us to speak about absence of tendencies for action against the background of dissatisfaction with the position in society: in drawings the experience of fear (characteristic drawing of eyes) is evident enough.

In the drawings, there are often details indicating the presence of protective tendencies accompanied by fear and anxiety (drawing and darkening of contour lines). As a rule, the nature of hatching is angular, constrained, which denotes tension, withdrawal, and in some drawings, line pressure and the nature of hatching correlate with such traits as aggressiveness and persistence. The "incomplete sentence" technique does not reveal a clear pattern of preference for positive or negative indicators in this group.

In the systems of attitudes towards coworkers, work and relatives both positive and negative indicators are found. In relation to oneself and one's capabilities, the indicators are more often positive.

Thus, in this group on the background of the reduction of social inclusion and deterioration of adaptability there are some manifestations of aggressive character, a significant part of the characteristics of the systems of relations is expressed by negative indicators. The presence of anxiety, tension and worries is also noted.

3.1.2 Clinical and psychological characteristics of group 2

All patients in the second group (24 patients) also suffered from the paranoid form of schizophrenia, and the first exacerbation happened relatively long ago - from 5 to 10 years. In the whole group the disease had an average progredient course, and the formation of the defect occurred in all patients.   The leading syndrome in 58.3% (14 cases) was hallucinatory-paranoid, including Kandinsky-Clerambaut syndrome, in 33% (8 cases) - paranoid syndrome, in 8.3% (2 cases) - depressive-paranoid syndrome.

In 42% (10 patients) the disease had a continuous, remission-free course; in 58% (14 patients) there was a seizure-progenerative type of course.

The clinical picture of this group of patients is characterized by persistent systematic progressive delirium of persecution and physical affect. Pseudohallucinations and phenomena of mental automatism are less pronounced. Delirium, being the predominant symptom, remains predominantly interpretative (unlike hallucinatory delirium in the variant described above). Personality changes during this period reach considerable severity. Thinking and speech are deeply upset. Inadequacy of facial expressions and paradoxical emotional reactions are pronounced. The social relations are sharply broken. Delirium determines the patient's behavior and makes professional activities   impossible (although memory and professional knowledge is intact). Patients are hospitalized for long periods of time. Depressive-paranoid type of seizure. Slow progression without polar variations in affect. In the initial period there were diurnal fluctuations, melancholic depersonalization, delusions of self-destruction (self-importance). At the same time, there was a combination of depression at the onset, along with anxiety and progressively more attitudinal ideas. Manifestation of each attack was accompanied by delusions of self-blame, sleep disorders, agitation.

The clinical picture is complicated by the development of symptoms that go beyond the purely affective: delirium of perception of the environment, delirium of meaning, condemnation. At the development of a seizure the imagery of delirium increased, it became fantastic, phenomena of mental automatism, delirium of physical influence are noted, at the height of a seizure delirium of staging, illusions of doubles, Cotard syndrome developed.

In the case of the seizure-progressive course of schizophrenia, personality changes preceded the onset of delineated seizures and progressed in leaps and bounds ("steps") after one or (less frequently) each seizure.

The true onset of the disease usually occurred during childhood, when developmental changes in the form of a particular dysontogenesis, as well as the formation of a schizoid character structure, were detected. In several cases it was possible to establish connection of these features of development with the erased seizures arriving on age crises. The clinic of such erased seizures was nonspecific and had a distinct age coloring (fears, obsessions, motor restlessness, dysthymia, etc.). However, after them, schizoid personality loomed and developmental delay in the form of mental infantilism was noted. In most cases, signs of early onset of the disease could not be detected, schizoid personality changes remained indistinct, and the disease was revealed only in connection with the development of manifestation seizures.

The clinical picture of seizures of attack-progressive schizophrenia included affective disorders. There were also complex syndromes with obsessions, depersonalizing, psychopathoid (in particular, heboid), paranoid, hallucinatory-paranoid disorders. A wide variety of depression types are possible, but the more typical, circulatory-like ones occur either before the manifestation or after some other unfolding episode ("acquired" circularity). Depressions were dysphoric, hypochondriacal, often accompanied by reasoning ("resonant depression") or limited to a decline in activity, lethargy without a feeling of ennui.

Kandinsky-Clerambaut syndrome was accompanied by psychic automatisms of all variants, confusion, delusions of staging, false recognitions, separate migrating catatonic disorders, delusions of physical effects and psychic automatisms taking the leading place here, There remained pronounced psychic infantilism, passivity, emotional impoverishment, often cyclothymic-like swings of affect.

Syndromologically, this group is represented by a spectrum of hallucinatory-paranoid, paranoid, and depressive-paranoid syndromes.

The presence of hallucinatory-paranoid syndrome was detected in 58% (14 patients) of the selected group. This syndrome was characterized by hallucinatory delusional experiences. However, delirium developed, as a rule, earlier, and verbal hallucinations appeared on the background of unsystematized ideas of attitude, persecution, on the one hand feeding the content of delirium, contributing to its amplification and development, and on the other hand reflecting the facet of delirium. Hallucinatory monologue, imperative hallucinations were often observed. Delirium of persecution was noted more often, less often - had sensory character and was accompanied by affect of confusion, fear and anxiety. Among mood disorders heaviness of mind and depression dominated. Pseudo-hallucinations were manifested by "voices" commenting on the patients' actions. With dominance of rank 1 symptoms according to C. Schneider, we regarded this syndrome as Kandinsky-Clerambaut syndrome.

Paranoid syndrome was noted in 33% (8 examinees of this group). The leading clinical manifestations characteristic of this syndrome were diffuse suspicion, which began as "delusional knowledge". As the pathological process progressed, the distorted assessment and processing of external events in these patients developed into delusions of persecution, values, and attitudes. No hallucinatory, pseudo-hallucinatory phenomena were revealed. The patients noted that "everything around is rigged, filled with a special meaning, and has a direct relation to them".

Some monotony of mental processes, decrease of physical and intellectual productivity was noted. Increased fixation on one's sensations, emotional detachment from the environment, and inability to critically assess one's condition were noted.

Among the rank 1 symptoms according to C. Schneider, the most frequent ones in the selected group of patients were:

- commentatory auditory hallucinations detected in 58% (14 patients) of this group;

- sounding of own thoughts was noted in 48% (12 patients);

- delusional imagination was observed in 64% (15 patients);

- somatic hallucinations were observed in 17% (4 patients);

- impact on thoughts, impact on feelings in 58% (14 patients);

Thus, peculiarities of the clinic in patients of Group 2 are characterized by: hallucinatory-paranoid; paranoid; depressive-paranoid symptoms. Among the rank 1 symptoms, the following predominate: commenting auditory hallucinations; sounding of own thoughts; somatic hallucinations; ideational and sensory automatisms.

Results of the psychological study of the 2nd group

Patients in this group had low values on the "introversion-extroversion" scale (2-6, "introvert") of the Eisenk test, which were somewhat lower compared to Group 1, i.e. introversion was stronger, thus, along with reticence, insociability, social passivity and inclination toward self-analysis, one can speak about an increase in difficulties in interpersonal communications, inner peace orientation, restraint, and remoteness. Pessimistic tendencies prevail in the character traits. Slightly elevated indices on the scale "neuroticity" (12-20) denote insecurity, tendency to irritability, unevenness in contacts with people. Also, these scores reflect inadequately strong reactions in relation to stimuli that provoke them. At the same time, some patients in this group had high scores on the neuroticism scale combined with high scores on the extraversion scale, indicating impulsiveness, irascibility, and excitability.

The analysis of drawings (the test "Nonexistent animal") shows the presence of fear of activity, tendencies for reflection which in a combination to the details frequently found in drawings (horns, claws, needles) specify the presence of unexpressed aggressive tendencies of both defensive and spontaneous nature. These tendencies are also indicated by the thematic nature of the animals (predominantly "threatening") and the large number of characteristic angles in the drawings. The doubled lines encountered in drawings are an indication of apprehension and suspiciousness of patients in this group.

In some drawings, there are mechanical parts, buttons, and keys built into the body of the "animal" that imply controlling the "animal" from the outside and denote the presence of "estranged" parts inside the "organism".

The "incomplete sentence" technique is dominated by negative indicators of relationship systems (work, loved ones, co-workers). Positive indicators are manifested mainly in relation to oneself and one's capabilities.

In addition, during the "incomplete sentence" test, elements of resonance were noted, and some answers were pretentious in nature.

Thus, in this group, along with an increase in social distance, an increase in introversion, and an orientation toward the inner world, an increase in internal tension, an increase in suspiciousness, and an increase in latent aggressive tendencies are noted. Besides, various nuances of test performance indicate an increasing manifestation of schizophrenic defect (pretentiousness, resonance, the presence of alienated parts and the idea of external influence). It should also be noted that increased tension and discordant tendencies are determined by the unfavorable presence of opposite tendencies-increase of affectively charged ideas and aggressiveness and at the same time decrease of connection with the external world and loss of even potential possibilities of their expression.

3.1.3 Clinical and psychological characteristics of group 3

All patients in the third group (30 patients) also suffered from the paranoid form of schizophrenia, with a disease duration of more than 10 years. The disease in this group of patients also had a medium progredient course, and the defect had long since formed (mostly of the mixed type) and came to the forefront in relation to the productive symptomatology. The leading productive syndrome in 60% (18 cases) was hallucinatory-paranoid, including Kandinsky-Clerambaut syndrome, in 30% (9 cases) - paranoid syndrome, in 10% (3 cases) - depressive-paranoid syndrome.

In 53% (16 patients) the disease had a continuous, remission-free course; in 47% (14 patients) there was a seizure-progenerative type of course.

In this group of patients (if the disease is not stabilized), delirium (persecution and influence) becomes global. The phenomena of mental automatism up to pronounced delirium depersonalization (the patient does not belong to himself, he is controlled by extraneous forces) become much more noticeable. Delirium loses strict systematization - speech becomes disjointed and includes unusual and peculiar word formations (neologisms). In some cases, speech disintegration is observed while the intonational structure and formal grammatical structure of a sentence remain. At external prompting (in the presence of the listener), some patients spoke non-stop (monologue symptom). Unlike speech incoherence in acute conditions, externally ordered behavior was preserved. Such patients have sharply expressed regression of behavior (unkemptness, gluttony, loss of general human skills).

The described clinical picture, accompanied by deep emotional devastation, loss of individual personality traits, indicates that the process reaches the final state, and deficit disorders come to the fore.

Some patients in this group had a residual hallucinatory-paranoid state. It was characterized by a combination of features of pronounced mental defect with persistent residual hallucinatory-paranoid symptoms. There was a simultaneous coexistence of delusions of persecution, influence, and grandeur. However, the delirium was devoid of systematization, appeared in the form of dry, frozen verbal formulas on the background of emotional smoothness, sullenness, autism.

Thinking had a paralogical character with elements of discontinuity. The background of mood depended on the contents of experiences. In the clinical symptomatology - in the presence of hallucinatory-paranoid disorders, emotional desolation and disconnected thinking were observed.

An attack-like course of the disease was characteristic. The basis of symptomatology at the moment of examination made asthenic changes in the form of reduction of energetic level of the personality. These patients were characterized by reduction of productive, purposeful thinking and smoothing of emotional modulations, indifferent attitude towards relatives. Such states are traditionally designated as - "reduction of energy potential" (Conrad), "dynamic desolation" (Jantzarik), "hypotonia of consciousness" (Berce), etc.

Apathetic-abulatory condition was noted in 8 patients (27% of patients in this group). Characteristic for this condition were - emotional dullness, flattening, poverty of internal experiences, indifference to what is happening. Some patients had hallucinatory-paranoid inclusions, which lost their relevance.

We should also note the presence of first-rank symptoms in patients in this group - thus, delusional imagination, auditory, contradictory, mutually exclusive hallucinations; comorbid auditory hallucinations come to the fore.

However, the clinical picture was dominated by negative symptoms in the form of emotional impoverishment, abrupt thought disorders (in 89% - 27 patients in this group), reduction of energy potential (in 47% - 14 patients in this group) and emotional inadequacy (in 89% - 27 patients in this group).

Thus, our distinguished group is characterized by the following clinical features:

- negative, deficit symptomatology predominates, reflecting remote stages of the course of schizophrenia;

- productive disorders lose their relevance, are reduced.

In this group, with moderately high scores on the neuroticism scale, some patients had high scores on the extraversion scale, indicating impulsiveness, irritability, irascibility, possible manifestations of aggression, and explosive personality traits. However, the index "introversion - extraversion" was very low (1-5, "introvert", "superintrovert"), lower than in Group 2.

Thus, along with reticence, restraint and focus on the inner world, the indicators of this group also indicate fear of contact, social alienation, a peculiar approach to interpersonal relations, elements of autism and emotional coldness.

The elevated level of the "neuroticism" scale (mean value) reflects the difficulties of adaptation. In addition, it should be noted that the reliability of some results of this test in this group may not always be recognized as high due to the elevated values of the "sincerity" scale (4-6 points, "situational sincerity"). This indicates the intention of part of the patients in this group (27% of the total group) to give socially desirable answers and is indicative of the closeness of the subjects and their negative attitude towards the study.

In drawings of the "nonexistent animal" of this group, the distinguishing features were low productivity, emotional impoverishment, emptiness (a drawing of several hardly visible lines, an empty circle), elements of fragmentation ("animal" in the form of an eye - "observer").

In addition, pseudo-symbols were used in the drawings, elements of graphic stereotyping were often encountered. During performance of the task, a decrease in criticality, a stable orientation towards internal evaluation criteria, and an inability to master instructions were also noted (instead of a non-existent animal with a non-existent name, a drawing of a cat with the name "cat2"). Therefore, in some of the projective drawings the analysis was impossible because of the lack of content, and such drawings were analyzed similarly to the consideration of graphic products in the pictogram technique.

In the "incomplete sentence" test, the manifestations of crude formality ("I think that my father... is my mother's husband") should be noted.

Elements of verbal stereotyping (socially desirable one-type, formal answers) were noted in a significant part of the patients. The other part of the patients assessed the most part of personal attitude systems mainly negatively.

Thus, in this group together with the orientation on the inner world, emotional aloofness and autism one can note manifestations of negativism, closedness in relation to the outer world in general and to the testing procedure in particular. These traits are noted on the background of decreased productivity, emasculatedness, manifestations of resonance and intellectual decline to the level of crude formality, which, in turn, emphasizes the increase of schizophrenic defect.

3.1.4 Clinical and psychological characteristics of group 4

The patients in this group (7 persons) suffered from simple low-progressive (according to the old classification - lethargic) form of schizophrenia with continuous type of course. Of them 4 persons had neurosis-like form, and 3 persons - psychopath-like form of schizophrenia. Distribution by syndromes: 14.3% depressive- hypochondriac, 28.5% psychopathoid-like, 2.2% senestopathic, 28.5% asthenic syndrome.

This schizophrenia is characterized by a very slow course and a gradual accumulation of personality changes, never reaching profound emotional devastation.

The disease occurred more often in adolescence. Initial symptoms were sharpening of pubertal traits of psyche with strengthening of emotional instability, irritability, oppositional attitude to relatives, reflexion. Along with these there was autistic detachment, asthenization, especially evident in mental activity, propensity to abstract meditations and general decrease in the range of interests. The subtlety of affective reactions was lost. On this background there appeared persistent neurosis-like disorders: obsessive, astheno- hypochondriacal and depersonalizing, hysteria-like, supercenic.

Intensity of these disorders fluctuated during many years, gradually they began to dominate in a clinical picture and defined a developed (manifest) stage of illness. In some patients one neurosis-like disorder prevailed, but in many patients various symptoms were combined.

Results of the psychological study of group 4

Patients in this group according to Eisenk's test results, with moderately high, on average for the group, indices on the "neuroticism"   scale (at the level of 15-18 "potential discordant" and 19-22 "discordant"), no marked tendencies were revealed on the "introversion-extroversion" scale. In the group, indicators of the entire range of this scale were expressed in the middle register (without extreme values) - "introvert", "potential introvert", "ambivert", "potential extrovert", "extrovert".

Thus, some increase in the "neuroticism"   index in this group reflects such traits as sensitivity, anxiety, some emotional instability, and a tendency to be painfully distressed by failures and upset by trivialities.

The analysis of graphic production (test "non-existent animal") is based on revealing the features repeated in most drawings of the subjects, which allow to reveal the following personal features of patients at the moment of test performance: low self-esteem, indecisiveness, absence of tendency to self-assertion, expressed tendency to reflection and reflection.

Details of drawing of many drawings reflect such features as sensuality, verbal activity, ease of occurrence of fears and fears. Often there are elements indicating dissatisfaction with oneself, doubts about one's own rightness, regrets about what has been done, a critical attitude to missed opportunities and one's own indecisiveness.

At the same time it is necessary to note a great variety of drawings and difficulty of definition of general features (each of allocated features is met no more than in half of drawings) of all patients in this group which can specify on affinity of this group to normative, i.e. to group of healthy, in which all types of characters and conditions are equally enough presented and in which, therefore, single general features for all examinees cannot be allocated.

In the "incomplete sentence" test, the system of attitudes towards oneself and one's capabilities is characterized by both positive and negative indicators. Attitudes towards family, relatives and co-workers are mostly expressed by positive characteristics. Fears and concerns, as well as statements related to guilt, are sufficiently detailed.

Thus, according to the results of data processing of the battery of tests we can speak about high expression in patients of this group of such indicators as low self-esteem, indecision, anxiety, propensity to experience failures, heightened reflexion at sufficient social involvement and, mainly, positive system of relations with the surrounding world.

3.1.5 Clinical and psychological characteristics of the control group

Patients referred to the control group (46 patients) had the following diagnoses: reactive psychosis - 2 patients (5%) and psychopathies - 44 patients (95%). The leading syndrome in patients with reactive psychosis was hallucinatory-paranoid, and the following types of psychopathies were observed among the patients with reactive psychosis: excitable - 4 patients (8.7%), hysteroid - 5 patients (10.9%), schizoid - 2 patients (4.3%), paranoid - 4 patients (8.7%), unstable - 20 patients (43.5%), mosaic - 9 patients (18.6%).

Reactive psychoses were influenced by mental trauma that caused fear, anxiety, apprehension, resentment, longing, or other negative emotions.

Mechanisms of emergence of reactive states in the aspect of the doctrine on higher nervous activity can be explained as a disruption of normal cortical activity as a result of overstretching of irritable and inhibitory processes or their mobility. A strong psychotraumatic effect is caused by an "error" in the irritant and inhibitory processes (concealed grief, repressed anger, etc.).

Simultaneously with changes in higher nervous activity there are humoral shifts (increased release of adrenaline, hyperglycemia, increased blood clotting, etc.) that occur during reactions of fear, anger. At high emotional stress there is a restructuring of the internal environment of the body, associated with the functions of the pituitary-adrenal system.

The main symptoms in the clinical picture of psychogenic paranoia were ideas of persecution, attitude and physical affect against a background of pronounced fear and confusion. The content of delusions reflected a psychologically traumatic situation and everything that happened was subjected to delusional interpretation and acquired special meaning. Besides delusions of persecution, relation and physical influence, the patients had abundant both auditory and visual hallucinations and pseudohallucinations; the affect of fear dominated in the status.

Diagnosis of reactive paranoids had the following basic criteria: situational conditionality, specific, imaginative, sensual delirium, connection of its content with a psychotraumatic situation and reversibility of this condition with changes in the external environment.

The acute paranoid reaction occurred suddenly, sometimes without any precursors. It is an acute figurative delirium of persecution and unusually sharp fear affect. At the height of the fear affect there was a disturbance of consciousness followed by partial amnesia for a specified period of time. Such paranoids were usually short-lived and when the patients were removed from the given environment the delirium disappeared and criticism of the psychosis appeared.

Clinical manifestations of psychopathies were characterized by the following features. Individuals suffering from these diseases were characterized by a disharmonious personality complex, which led them to disorders of social adaptation. Psychopathic manifestations were total and stable. Psychopathic disorders were not observed in this group. The most expressed disorders in psychopathic personalities were observed in the emotional-volitional sphere. Emotional reactions in some of them were characterized by excessive expression, with violent outbursts of anger and aggressive behavior, in others - with feelings of inferiority, anxiety, fear.

<u>Hysterical type</u>. Most typical for these patients was a desire to appear in their own opinion and in the eyes of others as a significant personality, which does not correspond to the real capabilities. Outwardly the specified tendencies are shown in aspiration to originality, demonstration of superiority, passionate search and thirst for knowledge of others, hyperbolization and coloring of their experiences, theatricality and show off in behavior, posturing, falsity, propensity to deliberate exaggerations, the actions calculated on external effect. Their emotions are bright, boisterous in their external manifestations, but extremely unstable and superficial, their excitement and grief are unstable and shallow. A characteristic feature of hysterical personalities - self-centeredness. Those of them, whose prevalence was not a thirst for recognition, and fantasy and mendacity, were called pathological liars, pseudologues, mythomaniacs. To draw attention to themselves, they told extraordinary stories, in which they assigned to themselves the role of protagonists, spoke about inhuman suffering they endured, could impress others with unusual manifestations of some disease with demonstration of seizures, fainting, did not stop at false accusations or self-talk (for example, ascribed to themselves the crimes which they did not commit), etc. Hysterical subjects are significantly more influenced by direct impressions than by those perceived through the second signal system, i.e., logically meaningful impressions. The psyche of such persons is extremely immature and bears the features of infantilism.

Excitable (epileptoid) type. Psychopathic individuals of this type live in constant tension with extreme irritability, reaching the point of rage, where the strength of the reaction does not match the strength of the stimulus. Usually after an outburst of anger the patients regret what has happened, but under the right conditions they do the same again. High insistence on others, unwillingness to reckon with their opinion, extreme egoism and selfishness, resentfulness and suspiciousness are typical for them. In some cases, in addition to pronounced explosiveness, a significant place is occupied by viscosity of affect, pedantry, thoroughness, sluggishness and tenacity of thinking. Attacks of a mood disorder (dysphoria) in the form of malicious melancholy, sometimes with fear are possible. These people are prone to conflict, uncooperative, stubborn, overbearing, petty nagging, demanding obedience and submission.

Paranoid type. The main feature of this psychopathy is the tendency to form super-valued ideas that influence the behavior of the individual. These are people with narrow and one-sided interests, distrustful and suspicious, with heightened ego and self-centeredness, stubborn in defense of their beliefs, sullen and vindictive, often rude and tactless, ready to see everyone as an ill-wisher.

Such properties, as well as narrow-mindedness and one-sidedness of thinking, low mental plasticity causing fixation on the same thoughts and affects, persistence turning into stubbornness, induced such subjects to continuous conflicts, harassment, struggle with imaginary enemies. Their thinking on the one hand is immature, childish, with a tendency to fantasies, and on the other hand, with a tendency to resonance. Accordingly, poor ideas and one-sided thinking determine affective life by one-sided and strong affects. They are men of action, pushy, uncompromising, humorless, straightforward in judgment, arrogant, and extremely self-righteous.

The content of super-valuable ideas may seem to be a reassessment of one's personality with a desire to be inventive, reformative. In contrast to delusional ideas, super-valuable ideas have sufficient life substantiation. They are more closely connected with real events and are more concrete in content. However, theoretical constructions usually grow out of one-sidedly noted and perceived facts, logic of thinking is subjective, judgments are erroneous. Failure to recognize the merits and merits, psychopathic personality leads to confrontation with others. Persuasions, threats, requests he is not amenable to.

Failures do not stop, but only add strength for further struggle. Activity, stenicism and persistence "in the struggle for justice" is manifested in endless letters, complaints, litigations and legal proceedings. Very high affective tension and at the same time lack of warmth of soul are characteristic.

<u>Schizoid type.</u> Psychopathic personalities of schizoid type were characterized by pathological reticence, secrecy, detachment from reality, autism. Absence of internal unity and consistency of mental activity as a whole, whimsicality and paradoxicality of emotional life and behavior, absence of synthonality were peculiar to them. The emotional disharmony of these persons is characterized by the so-called psychoethical disproportion, i.e. combination of hypersensitivity (hyperesthesia) and emotional coldness (anesthesia) with simultaneous estrangement from people ("tree and glass"). Such a person is detached from reality, inclined to symbolism, complex theoretical constructions. His will is extremely one-sidedly developed, and emotional discharges are often completely unexpected and inadequate.

Due to their insularity and impaired contact with reality, it is perceived very subjectively and inaccurately, as "in a crooked mirror". These persons have no emotional resonance with other people's experiences, it is difficult for them to find an adequate form of contact with others. In life, they are usually referred to as originals, weirdos, oddballs, and eccentrics.

The quirkiness of their intellectual activity is manifested in a special generalization of facts, formation of concepts and their combinations, logical combinations, unexpected conclusions, resonant reasoning and tendency to symbolism. Their judgments about people are usually categorical and prone to extremes. These people are biased, distrustful, and suspicious.

They are uncontrollable in their work, because they often work based on their own perceptions, then they are monotonously active. They in a number of areas where originality of thinking, artistic talent, special taste are required, they can under appropriate conditions achieve a lot.

The emotional life of schizoid personalities is also poorly understood and unusual. They are capable of subtle feelings and emotional responses to imagined images. Pathos and readiness for self-sacrifice. For the sake of the triumph of abstract concentrations of the universal order are combined in them with an inability to understand and respond to the emotions of loved ones and others of the real environment. Attention is selectively directed only to matters not of interest to them, beyond which they show absent-mindedness and lack of interest. They have a strong stubbornness and negativism in addition to their credulity and credulity. Passivity, inactivity in solving everyday problems is combined with an entrepreneurial spirit in achieving particularly significant goals for them. Their movements are peculiar, angular, lacking harmony and plasticity. Motor disorders were manifested in unnaturalness, affectation of facial expressions and gestures, caricatured gait, pretentiousness of handwriting, speech and intonation.

Depending on the prevalence of the hyperaesthetic or anesthetic component, there are sensitized and cold schizoid personalities. Sensitive persons, along with paradoxical and bizarre mental life, are highly vulnerable and sensitive, mistrustful, inclined to attribute much of what is going on around to their own account without justification. Inactive, shy, withdrawn and unsociable, they prefer solitude, entirely go to himself in his fantasy world. Such individuals do not have a sense of sympathy and love, empathy, the concept of duty and patriotism. They are cold, cavalier and often cruel. In other cases these traits of schizoid psychopathy are combined with expansiveness, increased but one-sided and pedantic activity. The orientation of volitional efforts is often determined not by the interests of society, but by obscure inner impulses related to the content of supervalued constructions.

Unstable type. Instability of mental life of psychopathic personalities of this type is caused by their increased subordination to external influences. They are weak-willed, suggestible and compliant people who easily fall under the influence of the environment, especially bad ones. Realization of motives, desires and aspirations is determined not by internal goal settings, but by random external circumstances. Alone, they are bored, looking for society, in accordance with external stimuli easily change their plans, forms of behavior and occupation. Induced and unwilling, they often get drunk, use drugs, violate work discipline, become wasteful, gamblers, swindlers, etc. Under favorable social conditions they acquire positive work attitudes. However, the instability of their psyche determines the rapid transition from inspiration to laziness, sloppiness and disorganization. They constantly need control, encouragement and correction of behavior.

Results of a psychological study of the control group

Examination of the patients of this group according to Eisenk's test revealed high (more than 12 in 75% of cases) scores on the "neuroticism" scale, and high scores on the "extraversion" scale. High indices on the scale "extraversion" (20-23 points) characterize individual-psychological orientation of the patients of this group to the world of external objects and reflect sociability, impulsiveness, straightforwardness of judgements, orientation on external estimation, irascibility, propensity to risky actions. In cases of combination with high scores on a scale "neuroticism" the characteristic features are heightened excitability, abruptness, interruptedness of actions, force, unbalance, bright expression of emotional experiences. In the character of drawings (the technique "Unknown animal"), such features as high self-esteem, tendency to activity and realization of one's intentions, tendency to self-assertion are revealed in patients of this group. In many drawings, signs interpreted as egocentrism (location of the figure "full-face") are noted. In addition, in the majority of drawings the analysis reveals such characteristics as interest in information, importance of opinions about oneself. Details denoting demonstrativeness and impulsiveness in decision-making are frequent and signs of aggression (as a rule, spontaneous, rather than defensive) are also encountered. Emphasis of sexual attributes (udders, nipples, etc.) is not uncommon. The drawings have high general energy (a high number of details, "generous depiction"), which reflects high productivity.

According to the results of the "incomplete sentence" technique, it is possible to conclude that almost all patients in this group give extended, emotionally rich endings to sentences. As a rule, patients positively characterize themselves, their capabilities, and their past and future.

Negative characteristics of relations with parents, relatives, coworkers (especially in relation to superiors) were frequent. The system of relations was characterized as indifferent in the case of completion of sentences about fears and worries, as well as about guilt.

As a whole the received results specify high social involvement, excitability, impulsiveness, bright expression of emotional experiences, high productivity of thinking processes. The system of emotional attitudes in patients of this group represents a full spectrum of characteristics with an accent on positive in relation to the self and own possibilities.

Conclusion

Comparing the results in groups 1, 2, 3, 4 on the background of the control group, we may note two basic tendencies: on the one hand, from group 4 to group 1, 2, 3 there is an increase of social distance, inner peace orientation, emotional coldness and autization; on the other hand, from group 4 to group 3 in the same direction there is an increase of negativism, strengthening of internal aggressive tendencies, on the background of the schizophrenic defect expression growth. At the same time, in group 3, the expression of the signs of direct aggressive tendencies decreases due to the intellectual decline, emotional impoverishment and reduction of the energetic potential.

Thus, the increasing schizophrenic defect begins to play a "compensatory" role and decreases the expression of aggressive tendencies during test performance in group 3 can denote an increase in negativism towards the procedure itself as compared to other groups.

The permeability of nerve cell membranes increases, proteins get out of the cell, into the bloodstream, thus contact with the lymph and the formation of antibodies there, i.e. increase immunity.

The activity of lymphocytes in schizophrenia has been shown to be 2.4 p higher than in healthy individuals.

The appearance of anti-brain antibodies and sensitized neutrophils in the blood can be regarded as a stage of neurosensitization of the body due to the deployed destructive processes in the brain tissues.

Antigens act on CNS in an excitatory way both directly and indirectly through histamine. Histamine realizes the effect of antigens on tissues and cells of the histiocytic reticuloendothelial system.

It may be that piling up of biogenic amines, primarily histamine, leads to increased penetration of the GEB and contributes to the release of brain antigens into the cerebrospinal fluid and blood. Increased levels of N-CAM may be associated with cellular remodeling or possible degeneration of some cellular components of certain brain regions.

An increase in N-CAM may also be an indicator of enhanced synaptogenesis as a response to brain damage.

Impaired N-CAM content may be secondary to altered synaptogenesis or neuronal plasticity in schizophrenic patients.

The formation of autoantibodies can cause secondary pathological changes; these antibodies are considered autoaggressive.

The autoantibodies to neurospecific cytoskeleton proteins and to the adhesion molecule that we detected may appear as a result of impaired self-recognition mechanisms by the immune system. Neurofilament proteins are members of an extensive family of intermediate filament proteins. N-CAM is a member of the immunoglobulin family of adhesion proteins. The triplet of neurofilament proteins share common, cross-reactive, antigenic determinants with intermediate filament proteins of other histotypes. A similar situation is observed for N-CAM.

The emergence of "forbidden" clones of lymphocytes that react with their antigens can be induced by a huge number of factors. In neuropsychiatric disorders, a disruption in the interaction between the nervous and immune systems may have a significant impact. Both systems use mutually influencing mediators that regulate the functional response of cells to external stimuli.

Intersection of regulatory pathways entails the occurrence of pathological situations, simultaneously, in the nervous tissue and in the immune system. This makes it difficult to identify both the causes of pathogenesis and secondary changes. It is possible that autoantibodies detected in the serum of schizophrenic patients play a role in neuropsychiatric pathologies. However, the very appearance of autoantibodies to neuronal antigens can be regarded as a remote consequence of synaptic abnormalities.

Neuropsychiatric disorders do not have an unambiguous classification, clear boundaries and symptomatology as of today. Obviously, elucidation of the causes, development of diagnosis, methods of correction and possibly fractions that bind autoantibodies. Similarly, in the membrane fraction - polypeptides N-CAM 140 and 180 kDa.

To date, there is mixed data on the presence of autoantibodies to CNS antigens in various pathologies of the nervous system. Immunoglobulins reacting with glial fibrillary acidic protein (GFAP) and S-100 protein have been found in the serum of patients with senile Alzheimer's disease and vascular dementia, but not in presenile Alzheimer's disease. Autoantibodies against GFAP are found in 30% of patients with inflammatory CNS disease and multiple sclerosis. At the same time, immunoglobulins to CNS proteins were detected in the cerebrospinal fluid of these same patients in only 1% of cases.

It was also found that autoantibodies of patients with vascular dementia have higher affinity to acidic fragments of degraded GFAP, but not intact one. The authors suggest that autoantibodies are not generated by a secondary immune response to soluble and degraded glial filament protein, which can penetrate through defects in the blood-brain barrier.

Such autoreactive immunoglobulins may appear as a result of dysregulated immune processes. It is possible that autoantibodies affect astrocytic function and dementia pathogenesis.

Circulating autoantibodies to glial filaments and neurofilaments have been detected that may be associated with autoimmune pathology
autism [97].

There is an alternative suggestion - defects in the blood-brain barrier make CNS antigens available to immunocompetent
cells. As a result, an autoimmune reaction to neurospecific antigens develops [106]. A significant increase in the number of reactive astrocytes by immunohistochemical methods has been observed in schizophrenia and dementia patients [187]. It should be noted that unlike normal astrocytes, reactive astrocytes are characterized by intense fibrillogenesis and cytoskeleton rearrangements [89].

Changes in N-CAM in synaptic endings have been found in schizophrenia. The authors attribute these changes to disturbances in the normal functioning of mature synapses [99]. Other authors note an increase in the soluble form of 120 kDa N-CAM in the CSF as a result of pathological turnover of cell adhesion molecules in the CNS in patients with psychiatric disorders [98]. Experimental models have been created based only on the study of specific proteins, their metabolism and interactions.

Summarizing the analysis of the immunological study, the following conclusions can be made:

- The present data on the presence of autoantibodies to neurospecific antigens in the sera of schizophrenia patients may be useful in the diagnosis of this disease.

- Changes in N-CAM levels are associated with abnormalities in cellular brain function, which may be a reflection of the pathological processes that occur in the brains of schizophrenic patients.

- The increased serum N-CAM content of schizophrenia patients may be associated with cellular rearrangements or possible degeneration of some cellular components of certain brain regions.

- Increased N-CAM content may be an indicator of increased synaptogenesis as an appropriate response to brain damage.

- Disruption in N-CAM content may be secondary to altered synaptogenesis or neuronal plasticity in schizophrenic patients.

- The obtained data are consistent with the study on the violation of the blood-brain barrier in patients with schizophrenia and, as a consequence, there is penetration into the blood of neurospecific antigens. This, in turn, may be a stimulus for the formation of B-cell clones specific to them.

- The formation of autoantibodies to neurospecific proteins can cause secondary pathological changes; these antibodies are considered autoaggressive.

- The technique of detecting N-CAM in blood serum can be recommended for introduction into the complex of diagnostic measures in patients with schizophrenia.

SECTION 4.

METHODOLOGY OF STATISTICAL PROCESSING OF RESEARCH RESULTS

The results of the study were subjected to mathematical processing by means of Mikrosoft Exel spreadsheets. We compared the following parameters of studied indicators of groups of schizophrenia patients with control group and among themselves: anxiety level, extra-introversion, psychoproduction, aggressiveness, social activity, frequency of exacerbations, quality of remissions, criticality, self-care, progredibility, dissimulation; attitude to self, to family, to past and future, fears of guilt, as well as serum reaction level of these patients to neurospecific proteins.

For the convenience of calculations in a unified system, all the features selected for statistical analysis were expressed in conditional units from -3 to +3. Immunological indicators for a more accurate calculation are expressed in conditional units from 0 to 10.

It was required to determine whether the results were statistically valid or invalid.

In order to find out the applicability of parametric methods of statistical processing in comparing the traits between groups, it was required to determine whether the distribution of indicators of different traits within each group is normal. For this purpose, the indicators of one trait should satisfy the following conditions:

- the standard deviation should be substantially smaller than the mean deviation,

- the variance value should be smaller than the standard deviation.

The standard deviation was calculated using the formula:

$$\textbf{Standard deviation} = \sqrt{\frac{\Sigma d}{n}};$$

where d is the deviation of each of the obtained values from the arithmetic mean;

Σ - amount;

n is the number of data.

The mean deviation was calculated using the following formula:

$$\textbf{Mean deviation} = \frac{\Sigma |d|}{n},$$

where Σ is the sum;

$|d|$ - absolute value of each individual deviation from the mean,

n is the number of data.

The variance is a statistical value that characterizes how much the individual values deviate from the mean value in a given sample.

$$S^{-2} = \frac{1}{n}\sum_{k=1}^{n}(x_k - \bar{x})^2$$

where S^{-2} is the variance,

n is the number of features;

$\bar{x}$ - is the average value in the sample;

x_k - particular values of the indicators in individual subjects,

Σ - amount.

The following trait parameters have normal distribution in the groups:

- Group 1: immunological reactions; attitude towards the future, aggression, social activity, quality of remission;

- Group 2: immunological reactions; attitudes towards oneself, towards the past, guilt, psychoproduction, dissimulation;

- Group 3: immunological reactions; attitudes towards the past, towards the self psychoproduction, aggression, progredient, dissimulation;

- Group 4: attitude towards the future;

- control group: aggression.

To all samples meeting the above conditions, we applied parametric methods of statistical processing - Student's t-test for independent samples. This is a parametric method used to test hypotheses about the reliability of the difference in the mean when analyzing quantitative data in populations with a normal distribution using the following formula:

$$t = \frac{M_1 - M_2}{\sqrt{\frac{s_1^2}{n_1} + \frac{s_2^2}{n_2}}},$$

where $\overline{M}_1$ is the mean of the first sample;

$\overline{M}_2$ is the average of the second sample;

s_1 is the standard deviation for the first sample;

s_2 is the standard deviation for the second sample;

n_1 and n_2 are the number of elements in the first and second samples.

If the value of and is less than 0.05, it means that the probability of error is less than 5% and the difference between the samples can be considered credible.

The following differences were significant:

- between groups 1 and 2: number and strength of neurospecific responses;
- between groups 1 and 3: number and strength of neurospecific reactions; aggressiveness;
- between groups 1 and 4: attitudes towards the future;
- between groups 2 and 3: number and strength of neurospecific reactions; attitude to the self, to the past, psychoproduction, dissimulation;
- between 1 and control groups: aggressiveness;
- between group 3 and the control group: aggressiveness;

We applied the nonparametric x2 "chi-square method to the remaining samples that did not meet the conditions of parametric methods.

The non-parametric x2 method does not require computing the arithmetic mean or standard deviation. Its advantage is that it only requires knowledge of the dependence of the frequency distribution of two variables; this allows us to find out whether they are related or, conversely, independent. This method has no limitations inherent to Student's method: it can be applied even in cases when the distribution is not normal and the samples are small.

The method consists in assessing how similar the distributions of empirical and theoretical frequencies are to each other. If the difference between them is small, then we can assume that the deviations of the empirical frequencies from the theoretical ones are due to chance. If these distributions are high enough, then it can be assumed that the differences between them are significant and there is a relationship between the effect of the independent variable and the distribution of empirical frequencies. The value of x2 is calculated using the following formula:

$$x^2 = \sum \frac{(\Theta - T)^2}{T} \, ,$$

where E is the empirical frequency,

T - theoretical frequency,

$\sum$ is the sum.

In this case, the differences between the parameters can be considered reliable when the x2 value is less than 0.005.

The following differences were significant:

- between groups 1 and 2: guilt, aggression, psychoproduction,

dissimulation, quality of remissions, criticism, attitudes towards the past, towards

future, to self, to family, social activity, frequency of exacerbations.

- between groups 1 and 3: psychoproduction, guilt, aggression,

dissimulation, criticism, attitude to the past, to the future, to oneself, progredentia, social activity.

- between groups 2 and 3: guilt, psychoproduction, dissimulation, quality of remission, attitude towards the past, towards the future, towards self, towards family, progredibility, self-care.

- between groups 1 and 4: guilt, progredentia, social activity.

- between 1 and control groups: aggression, social activity.

- between 2 and control groups: aggression, social activity.

- between 3 and control groups: aggression, social activity.

- between 4 and control groups: aggression, social activity.

- between groups 2 and 4: social activity.

- between groups 3 and 4: social activity.

This indicates that these groups differ significantly in these traits.

The following differences were not significant:

- between groups 1 and 2: progredensity.

- between groups 1 and 3: quality of remissions, attitude to family, frequency of exacerbations.

- between groups 2 and 3: aggression, criticism, social activity, frequency of exacerbations.

- between groups 1 and 4: aggression, psychoproduction, criticism, attitude to the past, to oneself, to the family.

- between 4 and control groups: anxiety.

This suggests that there are some similarities in these traits between these groups.

Comparison of some parameters did not require the use of calculations, because their values did not vary, numerical differences were clearly visible.

For example, the parameters expressed to a greater or lesser degree in the experimental groups that were completely absent in the control group were as follows: presence of neurospecific proteins in blood serum, psychoproduction, dissimulation, negative attitude towards oneself, to the past, to the future, low social activity, frequency of exacerbations, guilt, progessiveness, introversion.

The overall result of the significance of differences and similarities between the groups is shown in Table 4.1.

Table 4.1

Overall result of the significance of differences between the groups

	1и2	1и3	2и3	1и4	1iC	2iK	3iC	4iK	2и4	3и4
neurospecific proteins	+	+	+	+	+	+	+	+	+	+
aggression	+	+	-	-	+	+	+	+	+	+
psycho-products	+	+	+	-	+	+	+	+	+	+
dissimulation	+	+	+	-	+	+	+	-	+	+
remission quality	+	-	+	+	+	+	+	-	+	+
criticism	+	+	-	-	+	+	+	+	-	-
progredensity	-	+	+	+	+	+	+	+	+	+
self-service	+	+	+	-	-	+	+	-	+	+
social activity	+	+	-	+	+	+	+	+	+	+
anxiety	-	-	-	+	+	+	+	-	-	-
frequency of exacerbations	+	-	-	+	+	+	+	-	+	+
feeling of guilt	+	+	+	-	-	+	+	-	+	+
relation to the past	+	+	+	-	-	+	+	+	+	+
relation to the future	+	+	+	+	-	+	+	+	+	+
attitude	+	+	+	-	-	+	+	+	+	+
family attitude	+	-	+	-	+	+	+	+	+	+

"+" - the difference is significant,

"-" - the features have similarities.

Thus, in most cases the groups reliably differ from each other on these features, which is confirmed statistically.

SECTION 5.

RELATION OF CLINICAL, PSYCHOLOGICAL AND IMMUNOLOGICAL FACTORS IN SOCIAL ADAPTATION OF SCHIZOPHRENIC PATIENTS

5.1 Role of immunological factors in the course of schizophrenia

It has been suggested that an immunological approach to the study of schizophrenia runs through the "crossroads" of research on the role of the environment, including the possible influence of a hypothetical schizophrenia virus, and the importance of hereditary predisposition for disease development [121, 149].

The data presented and the opinions of various authors on the considered issues of schizophrenia etiopathogenesis show that neuroautoimmune processes arising in the organism of schizophrenia patients, both in connection with hereditary predisposition and in response to nonspecific effects from the external social environment, may be one of the possible points of contact between genetic and environmental, social and biological factors in the pathogenesis of schizophrenia.

Consequently, further progress of our knowledge about schizophrenia, including the study of the role of immunological processes in the etiopathogenesis of the disease, reveals a direct connection to the problem of the correlation between the social and the biological in human pathology, which is "one of the most important methodological problems of psychiatry" [118].

The one-sided emphasis on biological mechanisms and neglect of social conditions in the etiopathogenesis of schizophrenia reflects a narrowly biological approach in medicine, which leads to the biologization of the pathological process with a fatalistic understanding of the development and course of the disease as genetically predetermined and inevitable.

The opposition of the social and the biological, as well as the isolated study of them, ignoring one side of the other lead to a simplified, "linear" interpretation of the genesis of schizophrenia, split the human disease into biological and social parts, reducing mental phenomena to either the biological or the social, to the "two factor theory", which does not correspond to the dialectical understanding of their relationships in the human body, in its health and disease.

Attempts to solve the question of the role of hereditary or environmental factors in the etiopathogenesis of the disease, despite the productivity of individual results and their importance in the development of the teaching of schizophrenia, have led to an accumulation of contradictory and difficult to compare scientific data, to opposite one-sided views on the causes and pathogenesis of schizophrenia.

As quite rightly noted, "different authors understand differently the essence of this interrelation of the biological and social in medicine and pathology", in connection with which there are still discussions and disputes on various theoretical and practical issues in psychiatry [8].

In psychiatry, there is still a division of mental disorders into endogenous and exogenous, which "not without reason, raises serious objections" [19]. The insufficient development of the main methodological problem - the ratio of the social and biological in human pathology - explains the "far from perfect" results of one-sided biological and sociological studies in psychiatry [53].

The most important methodological prerequisite for solving the socio-biological problem in medicine is the dialectical and materialistic concept of the integrity of the complex structural and functional levels of the human organism, as well as the environment, without which "the existence of the organism is impossible".

Man as a social creature, which evolved from the animal, in a new quality acts as a certain integrity, a system of interaction between the biological and social levels of development. "The animal organism, noted I. P. Pavlov (1949), is a complex system consisting of an almost infinite number of parts connected both with each other and in the form of a unified complex with the environment.

Another important definition of living organisms is the system of their vital activity, their interaction and mutual equilibrium with the external environment. A living organism is an "open system" that is hourly and daily dependent on its living conditions [105].

On the peculiarities of interaction between social and biological in the system "organism - environment" it is said: "The integrity of the organism, the composition and interaction of its components act, thus, as a result of not only the external environment, fixed in heredity, but also the internal activity of the organism itself, its ability to adaptive changeability" [16].

It is necessary to take into account the "ring principle" of their interaction on the basis of human integrity, in which the social and the biological "mutually condition each other and pass one into the other", constituting a "system of interaction" [84, 133, 196]. The social conditioning of the systems and function of the human body will be different subsequently due to their evolutionary and structural differences. Moreover, the correlative role of social and biological factors differs at different stages of the ontogenetic evolution of man during his historical development. Therefore, a greater dependence of neuropsychic activity and its disorders on social conditions than on the physiological processes associated with the evolutionarily older somatic systems has been found [84].

Noting the interaction of biological and social factors in humans, it is said that social requirements make a significant and sometimes decisive correction in the physiological processes of the body and its individual systems, up to changes in reactivity in response to biological, mental and other stimuli [19].

Both human and human pathology are biosocial, and therefore it is incorrect to separate these two sides of the pathological process, both methodologically and medico-biologically [90, 106].

It is dialectically necessary to understand disease as "life constrained in its freedom", and not to reduce its definition to the biological or social. Therefore it is possible to agree only with such definitions of human disease in which both the social and biological aspects of it are distinguished [8].

Since the social essence of man in disease suffers as a single system with the prevalence of violations of one or another of its components, one or another "level of integration", the ratio of biological and social in human pathology should be considered as a structurally complex system, as a "disorder of the integral system organization", as a multistage process of interaction between damaging and protective-adaptive factors at the level of the integral organism in its relationship with nature and the social environment [36, 68].

The task of medical science is to study the dialectical interaction of social and biological factors in this holistic system [196].

The theory of causality in pathology means that all changes in the state of a living system are determined by the material influences of this system and environmental factors [133].

Disease, as a consequence, is not the result of external influence and not the result of "organismal correlations" only, but a specific refraction of the external in the internal [134].

Based on the dialectical interpenetration of the biological and social in man himself, the division of the causes of disease into external and internal is erroneous and, in fact, makes no sense. All diseases, including hereditary ones, were eventually formed, consolidated and transmitted from generation to generation during the active interaction of man as an organism and an individual with his natural and social environment [53, 107].

The founders of Russian psychiatry outlined a correct understanding of the relationship between social and biological factors in mental disorders. Thus, as early as V.P. Serbsky (1900) pointed to the "bad sides of civilization" as the cause of growth of mental diseases, considering heredity, trauma, poisoning and various acute and chronic somatic diseases as their direct causes.

Natural and social factors act on humans indirectly, through their biological adaptive mechanisms, Therefore, the widespread view claiming that all diseases are ultimately caused by environmental hazards and its main component, social conditions, is unlikely to be correct [53].

It is believed that a variety of pathogenic influences on humans cannot be realized outside the biological (physiological) processes of the body [29].

However, the role of social and biological factors in the origin and course of various mental diseases is not the same. At one pole of the long series of pathology of mental activity are pathological states and processes caused mainly by the action of biological factors (hereditary forms of oligophrenia, severe forms of endogenous and exogenous - organic psychoses). At the other pole are the states caused mainly by the action of social factors (reactive states and neuroses) [139].

It is argued that if in the etiology of the so-called endogenous diseases, primarily schizophrenia, as well as exogenous-organic mental disorders, the leading role belongs to factors of biological order, in the etiology of psychogenic reactions, neuroses, pathological personality development the main causative factor belongs to social, microenvironmental factors [90].

On the example of comparative analysis of neuroses and psychopathies the conclusion is made that the role of social factor in causing neuroses prevails and determines their occurrence; on the contrary, in psychopathies the leading in etiology and pathogenesis is the constitutional biological insufficiency [152].

Considering in this aspect psychogenic diseases, alcoholism, vascular neuropsychiatric disorders, the diversity and complexity of the interaction of social and biological components in the genesis of these mental illnesses, the ambiguous role and nature of the impact at different stages of the disease course are emphasized [118, 188].

A comparison of the genesis of two so-called endogenous mental diseases - schizophrenia and manic-depressive psychosis in pairs of identical and identical twins - has also shown that both hereditary and external (social) factors in different ratios play an important role in the development of both diseases [109].

Consequently, there is no reason to differentiate mental illnesses into endogenous and exogenous, biological and social. All of them arise as a result of the interaction of social and biological factors, acting in the emergence of various mental illnesses in unity and complex dialectical relations.

The correlation of social and biological in the pathogenesis of mental disorders should be considered from the recognition of the "unity of etiology and pathogenesis" [152].

Pathogenesis in its essence is a biological phenomenon, but this does not mean ignoring the influence of social factors on its mechanisms. Thus, pathogenesis in the system of medical cognition as a sociobiological mechanism of disease, which is determined simultaneously by natural and social factors, which allows to highlight the structure of "formed systems" and reflect the restructuring of functions and states of the human body [3].

As it turned out, many processes that outwardly look "purely" biological ultimately depend on social factors. This is also true for disorders of immunological reactivity, which play an important role in the pathogenesis of schizophrenia.

The immune system, designed to maintain the constancy of the antigenic composition of the organism, protection from alien genetic information and thereby ensure the constancy of the internal environment, is an extremely sensitive mechanism that quickly responds to relatively weak but evolutionarily unexpected factors (O.V. Baroyan, 1978). Therefore, the isolation of an internal factor, immunological reactivity, from the causal interaction does not mean ignoring other elements, including environmental factors [73].

Thus, the position on the unity and dialectical interaction of social and biological factors in the etiopathogenesis of disease is one of the fundamental methodological and scientific methodological principles that help to bring clarity to the direction of theoretical research and practical work in modern psychiatry.

At the same time, the role of social and biological factors is different in different mental illnesses and at different stages of their development, and their components are not identical. Therefore, psychiatry faces the task of specifically deciphering this formula, taking into account the nosological and clinical form of the disease [61, 90, 111, 152].

If a disease is a combined process of an adverse effect of the external environment and the organism's response to it, then the task of the researcher is to address both the analysis of environmental factors and the study of the organism's reactivity [155].

It is possible to reveal these features of interaction of internal and external, biological and social in etiopathogenesis of schizophrenia only on the basis of scientifically grounded system approach which main attribute is understanding of integrity of human vital activity, his health and illness.

5.2 General characteristics of the dynamics of immunological processes and their role in the pathogenesis of schizophrenia

The study of nonspecific defense components and immunological reactivity, neuroallergic and neuroautoimmune shifts in patients with schizophrenia is devoted to a large number of works. However, the use of different immunological tests for this purpose and the examination of selective groups of patients led to inconsistencies in the results obtained, which make it difficult to have a holistic view of the dynamics of non-specific protection indices and immunological reactivity specific to brain antigens. Since there are conflicting opinions and conclusions on the relationship between various immunological reactivity indices and the course of the schizophrenic process, there is still no unity of views on the role of these factors in the pathogenesis of the disease.

Considering also the regional peculiarities of the immunological status of patients with schizophrenia, it was assumed that the use of the epidemiological approach to the study of the immunopathogenesis of schizophrenia would allow to deepen the understanding of the correlation of changes in various parts of the immunological system of the patients' organism (indices of non-specific protection, neuroallergic and neuroautoimmune shifts) to determine their significance in the development of the disease [33, 72].

Results of the study of nonspecific defence indicators

The study of individual indices of nonspecific protection in schizophrenia has been conducted for a long time. Nevertheless, there is still no clarity about the patterns of fluctuations of nonspecific defense factors in the course of schizophrenia, the mechanisms leading to an increase or decrease in their content, and the significance of these fluctuations for the clinical disease. Opinions and conclusions of researchers regarding the dynamics of natural immunity factors in the course of schizophrenia are controversial: some emphasize low levels of nonspecific protection factors, regardless of the period of the disease course, others note their increase in connection with the improvement of mental condition, while others point rather to the opposite dynamics, namely, the increase of nonspecific immunological mechanisms during the exacerbation of psychosis and their decrease during remission.

As an indicator of cellular immunity, characterizing the T-system of lymphocytes, the development of delayed-type hypersensitivity was studied by skin-allergic reaction to common antigen (tuberculin) and anti-tissue serum. Functional state of humoral immunity, reflecting B-system of lymphocytes, was investigated by determination of level of immunoglobulins of classes M, U and A and complement in blood of patients.

Unequal activity was observed. T-cells in relation to tuberculin and anti-tissue immune serum. The drop in the activity of cellular immunity in relation to the antigens studied may be a consequence of the deficiency of a certain clone of T cells caused by the antithymic serum factor detected in schizophrenia [96]. At the same time, one cannot also rule out the fact that the observed selective decrease in the activity of T cells in relation to the antigen serum may be caused by a decrease in the total number of receptors on lymphocytes due to their blocking in the blood of patients by autoantibodies.

The functional state of B-lymphocytes in schizophrenia was investigated by a widespread method - determination of the content of immunoglobulins of different classes in the blood of patients. The literature data on the content of immunoglobulins in schizophrenia are extremely contradictory. According to the author of a literature review devoted to the study of immunoglobulin content in the blood of schizophrenic patients, the inconsistent results of some researchers seem to be related to the heterogeneity of clinical material [92].

It is noteworthy that when studying the content of immunoglobulins in the blood of patients, some authors have established a relationship between their dynamics and some other clinical parameters. Thus, a higher level of immunoglobulins of all classes is observed in schizophrenia compared to the examined healthy individuals and their relationship with the severity, duration of the disease and age of patients has been established [2]. Not only have immunoglobulin levels been found to increase in the blood of schizophrenic patients compared to those of practically healthy individuals, but also to normalize their levels without a marked improvement in the condition when desensitization therapy is used [48].

In contrast to these authors A. Amkraunt, G. Solomon et al. (1973), A. A. Sugerman et al (1982) observed no statistically significant difference in the content of immunoglobulins in schizophrenic patients and healthy individuals, as well as depending on a number of clinical parameters and the therapy being conducted.

There are data on the content of immunoglobulins of classes M, G and A in the blood sera of patients, depending on the period of the course of schizophrenia [114]. During exacerbation of psychosis, a significant increase in IgG compared to the remission period is determined. During remission, a higher level of IgM was detected compared to the period of exacerbation. The observed regularities in the dynamics of immunoglobulin of different classes during exacerbation and remission in schizophrenia reflect the relationship between the studied humoral immunity parameters and the course of the disease.

After that, the presence of competing ratios between IgG and IgA on the one hand, and IgM on the other, possessing not only different physicochemical but also biological properties confirms the possibility of active involvement of immunological mechanisms in the pathogenesis of schizophrenia. These proteins, different in their physicochemical, biological (functional) and antigenic properties, have "antigenic" activity, i.e., they contain antibodies of different specificity. Therefore, determination of immunoglobulin levels in the blood of schizophrenia patients during psychosis exacerbation and remission characterized not only the dynamics of non-specific humoral immunological reactivity, but also, apparently, indirectly indicated the synthesis of anti-brain autoantibodies belonging to different classes of immunoglobulins.

Considering the possibility of parallelism between the level of immunoglobulins of different classes and the content of specific antibodies, in the light of the obtained data, it can be assumed that in the blood of patients during exacerbation of psychosis the prevalence of anti-brain autoantibodies of type IgG and IgA with increased permeability across the blood-brain barrier and cytotoxic properties towards the brain structures [158]. It is possible that during the remission period, autoantibodies of the IgM type prevailed, which did not possess such a property and, apparently, were the evidence of auto-sensitization or performed a protective function. In addition to these two indicators of cellular and humoral immunity, to assess non-specific immunological reactivity, we determined the complement activity of blood serum, which is an important factor of immunological protection of the body. According to the definition of the World Health Organization, complement is "a system of normal blood serum factors, activated in a special way by antigen-antibody complexes, which then mediates a chain of various biologically significant events.

Studies on the structure of serum complement activity in schizophrenia are few, and their results are heterogeneous and contradictory.

The first robots were performed on small groups of patients, and in them there was no analysis depending on the phases of the disease. There is no consensus on the patterns of complement dynamics in the blood during exacerbation and remission. Some researchers have noted a decrease in complement activity in the blood during exacerbations of schizophrenia, while others, on the contrary, have observed a relative increase in complement activity during exacerbations of the disease.

Taking into account the possible correlation found in dysgammaglobulinum patients with neuroautoimmune processes and mechanisms of antigen-antibody coupling during their interaction with complement, which "in some cases contribute to the development of damaged nervous tissue as well as anaphylactic reactions, alteration of peripheral blood leukocytes of the sensitized organism under the action of brain antigens", the establishment of interrelation between the dynamics of immunological reactivity

parameters studied and those of humo

The complexity and variety of mechanisms of humoral autoantibodies with aggressive, protective and neutral properties or being a normal physiological system that coordinates homeostasis and performs a transport function in "clearing" the body of residual metabolic and catabolic substances can explain the possibility of detecting various autoantibodies in healthy people as well as in a number of pathological conditions and diseases [8]. The detection of autoantibodies to brain antigens in the organism of schizophrenia patients and their relatives has been proved by many authors and is beyond doubt, and ongoing research to establish the role of these factors in the pathogenesis of the disease is one of the important and independent directions of its biological basis study. Currently, there are contradictory views and concepts on determining the role of anti-brain autoantibodies in the mechanisms of occurrence and course of schizophrenia (P. Grabar, 1975). Exacerbation of psychopathological disorders in schizophrenia is accompanied by activation of T-system immunity in relation to antigens of brain tissue, while suppression of this neuroallergic reaction is observed during remission.

The course of exacerbation in patients with schizophrenia is accompanied by increased activity of T-system lymphocytes found in cellular hypersensitivity reactions of delayed type in relation to brain antigens, as well as anti-tissue antibodies. At the same time during this period there is an activation of humoral immunity, in particular the synthesis of immunoglobulins of classes G and A, as well as humoral complete hemagglutinating and incomplete anti-brain autoantibodies. These clinical and immunological correlations may indicate the active involvement of mechanisms of interaction between cellular and humoral neuroautoimmunity in the development of schizophrenia relapses.

In contrast, the course of schizophrenic remissions was accompanied by inhibition of these neuroallergic responses as well as increased synthesis of M immunoglobulins.

5.3 Role of clinical and psychological factors in the course of schizophrenia

The modern level of knowledge on clinical forms of schizophrenia proceeds from the principal proposition that not the psychopathological syndrome currently defined in a patient "in a cross section", but the stereotype of disease development that is clinically expressed in a regular variation of syndromes "in a longitudinal section", characterizes the quality of the pathological process and allows a new classification of the disease [174, 179].

The clinical forms selected on the basis of the type of course and progression of the process persist throughout the course of the disease, which is a reflection of their stability and confirms the validity of the existing differentiation of schizophrenia [108]. Therefore, almost all previously formulated hypotheses related to individual prognostic criteria and scales of the course of schizophrenia, which were based on the old principles of classifying schizophrenia forms, need critical verification and evaluation.

Only now are there opportunities to outline the prerequisites and main directions of successful studies of the course of the process using mathematical-statistical methods for scientifically grounded "longitudinal" prediction of schizophrenia. However, such studies of the course of schizophrenia are only just beginning [140].

This chapter presents the results of a complex multifactorial study of schizophrenia from the standpoint of a systematic approach to understanding the patterns of disease development using clinical and immunological material while taking into account the social characteristics of the patient and the role of the external environment.

It was expected that such a scientifically based systematic approach to the study of clinical forms of the disease would provide new data on the role of some clinical, biological and social factors in the formation and prognosis of the course of schizophrenia, which would allow us to critically evaluate the hitherto existing unilateral conceptions in understanding the causes of its clinical polymorphism.

5.4 Role of some clinical and biological factors in the shaping of schizophrenia

In   contrast to Kraepelin's notion of dementia praecox, which was identified with an incurable and completely unfavorable prognosis, the association of the prognosis of the disease with the nature of its onset and the denial of the prognostic value of individual symptoms have been established. The unfavorable prognosis is more often combined with the chronic development of the disease and clinical manifestations with clear consciousness [138].

However, R. Holmboe and C. H. Astrup (1957) cite the results of a long follow-up study of 255 patients with schizophrenia with an acute onset and report that they were unable to identify the disease either by features of the onset or by further course of the disease.

The prognostic value of the type of onset (acute, gradual) is variable and of limited value (119).

The impossibility of basing the prognosis in schizophrenia on individual psychopathological symptoms is confirmed by the current study of the course of different clinical forms of the disease [138].

For example, the results of an international exploratory study of schizophrenia in nine countries under the auspices of WHO showed that the only reliable criterion for adverse prognosis was emotional insufficiency, while all other manifestations of schizophrenia were not reliably predictive (Carpenter W. T., Bartko J. J., Straus J. S., Hawk A. B., 1978).

The prognostic value of many other clinical and biological criteria, such as the presence of exogenous harmful factors, age, gender, heredity, is considered controversial by various researchers.

Early age of onset of schizophrenia has been considered a sign of the severity and malignancy of the process and an unfavorable prognosis [63, 154]. However, on the other hand, it is known that the schizophrenic process can proceed relatively favorably at an early age [184, 185, 186]. In the remaining age groups, different disease outcomes are also possible, which indicates the lack of prognostic significance of this factor in the course of schizophrenia [12, 42, 40, 63, 99, 120, 121, 131, 174, 175, 176, 177, 179].

The literature on the impact of gender on the clinic and course of schizophrenia is also extensive and heterogeneous. Some authors report that the prognosis of schizophrenia is better in females than in males [82]. It is also noted that seizure-like forms of endogenous psychosis occur much more frequently in women than in men [178]. Other authors, studying the timing of clinical defect formation in schizophrenia depending on gender. They did not establish the influence of this factor on the prognosis of the disease [101].

At the same time, the results of studies conducted at the Institute of Psychiatry of the USSR Academy of Medical Sciences convincingly show that the age-sex factor undoubtedly affects the degree of progredibility within the main forms of schizophrenia [174, 109]. An epidemiological study of schizophrenia showed that in the subpopulation of patients who fell ill before the age of 17, there were almost twice as many men as women, and malignant schizophrenia in this subpopulation was found 3 times more often than in the subpopulation of those who fell ill after 17 [109].

There is also heterogeneous data in the literature regarding the role of the hereditary factor as a prognostic criterion for the course of schizophrenia.

Hereditary aggravation of schizophrenia has been found more often in families of patients with a continuous course of the disease [120, 186]. Other researchers have found a seizure-like or intermittent course of schizophrenia in hereditarily burdened patients [100, 109, 139, 141].

L. Brlenmejer-Kimling, S. Nicol (1986) observed recovery and relatively persistent remissions in a control group without hereditary aggravation, compared with patients with hereditary aggravation of schizophrenia.

In the absence of direct signs of schizophrenia, an indication of remitting illness in relatives indicated a good prognosis, especially in patients with the catatonic form of schizophrenia (Winocur G., Tsuang M. T.).

At the same time, it is pointed out that when "abnormalities of character in the past" are found in patients with schizophrenia, the prognosis of the disease as a whole is clouded [139]. Therefore, a number of contemporary works take into account not only manifest cases of the disease, but also the presence of abnormalities in family members. Studies carried out in this way have found that manifestation with a continuous course is less likely to occur in patients with psychopathic abnormalities as well as in the presence of similar abnormalities in close relatives [102].

The distribution of cases with features of the mental state of parents of schizophrenic children (manifest psychosis, sterile forms of psychosis, stenotic schizoidy, mixed schizoidy, schizoidy with persistent emotional defect, asthenic schizoidy, hyperthymic personality complex) differed significantly in the families of probands with unfavorable and relatively favorable forms of the disease [93].

It has been established that an unfavorable course of schizophrenia (short remissions, increasing disability) is accompanied by a pronounced hereditary burden and certain anomalies in the premorbid character: mistrustfulness, tendency to introspection, withdrawal, etc. [12].

A correlation has been found between the variant course of juvenile onset schizophrenia and the background against which the disease arose (hereditary burden), as well as the clinical features of the initial stage of disease development [187].

An unfavorable course of schizophrenia under the influence of various exogenous factors has been noted; at the same time, a favorable influence of the same exogenous factors has been found [11, 113, 116, 127, 185].

It has been emphasized that the influence of various external harms (psychogenias, infections, etc.) on the occurrence of a psychotic outbreak in recurrent schizophrenia compared to other forms of schizophrenia   is particularly common (174).

On the basis of the materials of epidemiological research it was also noted that in the depressive-paranoid variant of periodic schizophrenia, the presence of exogenous harmfulness preceding the onset of the disease was observed in 69.5% of cases, while the same harmfulness in nuclear schizophrenia was observed in only 42.3% [37]. At the same time, it was found that in patients with schizophrenia, more than half of the seizures occurred due to some exogenous factors (alcoholism, psychotraumas, childbirth), i.e., somewhat more frequently than in recurrent schizophrenia [15].

The observations of many foreign authors suggest that the presence of provoking external factors has a rather favorable prognostic value, while in the absence of such factors, the course of the disease, as a rule, is more progenerous [110].

According to the data of follow-up examination of patients with schizophrenia M. Kato (1969) established that in case of recurrent course the onset of the disease was associated with psychogenic and somatic factors much more often (in 62.5%) than in other groups.

Consequently, a review of the literature suggests that there are contradictory data regarding the role of various clinical and biological factors in the prognosis of the course of schizophrenia, which points to the need for a differentiated study of them to comprehensively address the issue of disease formulation.

The possible relationship between the clinical forms of the course of schizophrenia and a certain complex of clinical and biological factors, namely sex, age, peculiarities of hereditary burdening of the patient, the age of the patient's mother at the time of birth, and the presence of provoking exogenous harmful influences, has been studied [114].

Given the previously established relationship between schizophrenia prevalence rates and age and sex characteristics of patients, it seemed appropriate to first analyze the possible influence of these clinical and biological factors determining prognosis duration: poor prognosis was predicted by lack of establishment of friendships, group activity, marital relationships and religious activity.

G. Huber, G. Gross, R. Schuttler (1975) also found no definite effect of social class affiliation on the long-term prognosis of schizophrenia.

In analyzing the predictive factors for the course of schizophrenia, it has been found that everything depends on the combination of disease progression, the patient's adverse situation and the influences experienced by the individual patient depending on how their environment affects them [147].

The works of some researchers analyze the prognostic value of educational and qualification level of patients on the course of schizophrenia. According to A. Farina, H. Garmezy, M. Becker (1962), G. M. Faibish, A. D. Pokorny (1972), higher educational attainment was negatively correlated with good outcome.

The theory of E. Zigler, L. Phillips (1961), on the contrary, was that social competence regarding professional educational achievement was favorable for the prognosis of schizophrenia. It was found that those in higher positions with a secondary or at least incomplete higher education were more likely to work, compared with workers who had not completed secondary education, who were concentrated in the non-working group (154).

Many authors have pointed to the prognostic value of the marital status of patients with schizophrenia and intrafamilial relationships on the course of the disease.

5.5 Role of some psychological factors in the course of schizophrenia

There is evidence in the literature on the effect of some social and environmental characteristics of patients on the long-term prognosis of the course of schizophrenia.

Theory A. B. Hollingsheat, F. C. Redlich (1958) referred to a direct relationship between prognosis in schizophrenia and social class. According to the authors, differences in the course of schizophrenia and the possibility of rehabilitation are due to the distribution of the disease between classes. Late detection of the disease, inadequate treatment, and difficulties in returning the patient to the family in the lower classes create conditions for the accumulation of "chronic patients".

There are also other observations (Faibish G. M. , Pokorny A. D, 1972) indicating that none of the studied socio-economic indicators of patients and their parents, including occupational level, showed any connection with the prognosis of schizophrenia. At the same time, according to these authors, past social behavior appears as a category most significantly long-standing patients in intensive care. In contrast, the duration and severity of the disease correlated with an increase in serum and cerebrospinal fluid IgG levels and low IgM levels.

Since the role of neuroautoimmune and neuroallergic shifts and their prognostic significance remain poorly understood to date, of particular interest are studies that have attempted to establish clinical and immunological correlations in relation to the efficacy of the therapy.

It has been noted that complement-binding autoantibodies to the brain antigen complex detected in the serum are usually accompanied by an unfavorable prognosis of the ongoing therapy [87].

It has been established in first-time inpatients that complete hemagglutinating antibodies to the brain have been detected in the acute onset and rapid increase of psychotic symptoms, which disappear with clinical improvement. In the absence of clinical improvement, disappearance of antibodies has not been observed (182).

Using the neutrophil damage reaction, the increased sensitivity of the patients' organism to brain antigens was established predominantly in the schizophrenia exacerbation state [101]. According to the author's data, a comparison of allergic reactions in cases of the episode course of schizophrenia showed that a favorable outcome very often coincided with the tension, high intensity of immunological reactions during the examination period. On the contrary, in patients with a continuous course, whose last exacerbation lasted up to 1.5-2 years and did not respond to therapy, the intensity of reactions was relatively low.

Studying the dynamics of autoimmune shifts (the content of brain antigens and anti-brain antibodies in blood serum) in patients with continuous forms of schizophrenia, it was found that a decrease in blood immunological activity is prognostically favorable with regard to the effectiveness of therapy, while high blood immunological activity usually corresponds to subsequent remissions of worse quality [44].

A simultaneous study of complement-binding and agglutinating autoantibodies in the brain revealed the peculiarities of their relationships during attacks and exacerbations of episode-type and continuous schizophrenia [45]. Seizures of intermittent schizophrenia were characterized by the early appearance of complement-binding autoantibodies in the blood, and by the later appearance of hemagglutinating autoantibodies at the height of the attack. In the period of remission formation hemagglutinating autoantibodies did not appear, and titer of complement-binding autoantibodies after some increase gradually decreased. The dynamics of anti-brain antibodies in continuous-progressive schizophrenia is characterized by their cyclic appearance and disappearance and does not show a close relationship with the severity of the therapeutic effect.

In the acute stage of schizophrenia, there is tension of neuroautoimmune processes and a simultaneous decrease in nonspecific reactivity [83].

There is also evidence in the literature of increased resistance to therapeutic interventions in schizophrenia patients born of immunogenetically incompatible ABO pregnancies, especially in patients with blood type A and mothers with blood type 0 [2, 54].

The found out clinical and immunological correlations in connection with immunocorrection in patients with schizophrenia confirm the important role of immunological factors in formation of therapeutic remissions.

The complex mechanisms of immunoreactive therapy were accompanied in schizophrenia by positive dynamics of immunological indices, which resulted in more complete remissions, shortened the period of hospitalization and created prerequisites for more effective psychopharmacotherapy.

As a result of this study, the possibility of suppressing autoimmune reactions in patients with persistent schizophrenia using anti-lymphocyte globulin has been established, which simultaneously significantly increases their reactivity to psychopharmacological drugs [164].

Normalization of immunoglobulin content and antiserum titer during immunostimulatory therapy of schizophrenia by administration of heterologous serum was noted, which was an objective indicator of treatment results according to the patients' mental state [76].

A.S. Vereshchagina (1980) found in cases of positive therapeutic effect during treatment of schizophrenia patients with cyclophosphan a statistically significant increase in complement levels a small decrease in beta-lysine levels and spontaneous blast-transformation reaction to brain antigen.

During treatment of patients with continuous schizophrenia with prodigiozan, quatioprine, and lidase against the background of traditional psychopharmacotherapy, a significant decrease in the titer of anti-brain antibodies and the level of neurosensitization of T-lymphocytes was observed, which was accompanied by an improvement in the mental status and the formation of better remissions [126, 161, 168, 169].

The possibility of obtaining a therapeutic effect accompanied by a normalization of the level of immunologic indexes was discovered when using the immunomodulator levamisole; as well as in the course of a course therapy with insulin and neuroleptics [2, 14, 32, 35, 77, 106, 143, 190, 191].

Thus, as can be seen from the above data, clinical, social and immunological factors simultaneously influence the effectiveness of therapy in schizophrenic patients.

Therefore, modern domestic as well as foreign psychiatry emphasizes the need for an integrated approach to treating patients with schizophrenia simultaneously at the biological and social levels, which may prove to be more fruitful as it expands the traditional areas of therapeutic intervention in mental disorders and substantiates the need for changes at different levels of the human "ecosystem" [5, 151].

5.6 Role of socio-biological and immunological factors in the establishment of remission in schizophrenia

A sufficiently high immediate effect of using modern active treatment methods of schizophrenia still does not allow obtaining stable long-term remissions [1]. Therefore, the search for methods of stabilization of therapeutic remissions, prevention of relapses and repeated hospitalizations should be considered the most important task in rehabilitation of patients with schizophrenia.

The belief that outpatient therapy with psychotropic medications is the main factor in preventing decompensation of the mental state in remission and reducing the quality of relapses is not shared by all researchers [85, 58, 124, 190].

Despite the widespread use of supportive therapy with psychotropic drugs in outpatient settings in schizophrenia patients, the duration of remission not only does not increase as one would expect, but also tends to shorten; as a result, patients are admitted to hospital more frequently than before the introduction of psychotropic drugs into psychiatric practice [1, 100, 102].

Other authors do not attribute decisive importance to maintenance therapy, but acknowledge a role of exogenous factors in the development of relapses and repeated hospital admissions.

According to one source, exogenous harms (psychogenia, alcoholism, overexertion, infections) preceded relapses in 47.2% of cases, and according to another, in 21% of cases [11, 64].

A further study of the causes and conditions favoring the occurrence of relapses and exacerbations found that in 22% of cases the onset of relapses is preceded by provocative exogenous harms (somatic diseases, psychogenias, childbirth, etc.), in 45% of cases relapses are due to discontinuation of psychotropic drugs or its errors and only 33% of cases the onset of relapses cannot be linked by any explicit factor [6].

Many foreign researchers who have studied the factors influencing the occurrence of schizophrenia relapses, give the leading role in the remission course to the patient's family [131]. In their opinion, the support of the family in which the patients stay, good living conditions, care, constant care and understanding on the part of their relatives have a significant influence here.

The cause of relapses and repeated hospitalizations, as found in the study, is primarily psychosocial factors (lack of support at home, unfavorable attitude towards the patient by relatives), while the severity of the disease, according to the authors, does not play any role.

However, there is another point of view, according to which a neutral environment is more favorable for ex-patients, as they get along worst with their wife, almost as badly with their parents, and best of all with distant relatives or strangers (146).

More detailed studies of patients' family life have found that poor prognosis in schizophrenia is not related to "high emotional involvement" of the family, but rather more to the nature of emotions expressed in the family in relation to the patient [147]. Researchers were able to show that the intensity of emotional involvement, reliably determined by repeated standardized questionnaires by the number of critical remarks they made about the patient. Nine months after discharge from the clinic, 58% of patients whose families had such high emotional "engagement" relapsed, while only 16% of patients from families with low emotional engagement relapsed.

A   similar conclusion was subsequently reached by other researchers, who also showed that one of the most significant predictors of schizophrenia relapse is the level of emotional reactions of the patient's relatives with whom he lives together and with whom the relationship is significant to him.

If in cases of negative emotional conditions in the family, relapses occur in 53% of patients, the risk of relapse increases up to 92%, when the patient does not take medication and restricting contacts with such relatives, remission periods are prolonged and relapses occur in only 15% of cases, which approximately coincides with the number of relapses in patients living in normal family conditions.

However, the preventive effect of supportive treatment was not effective for patients living in a family with high emotional expression, and conversely, the protective effect of supportive therapy was significant for patients living in a low emotional environment.

Convincing evidence of the important role of various environmental factors of the patient on the clinical parameters of the course of remission is the positive results of social and occupational therapy, allowing in a number of cases to prevent relapse of the disease [118, 133].

At the same time, there is no doubt that a combination of maintenance treatment with psychotropic drugs and psychosocial therapy has a more effective effect on the course of remissions.

Data from Moscow psychiatric hospitals are cited, according to which the duration of remission in patients engaged in psychotherapy and receiving medication is 1.5-2 times higher than in patients included in labor processes [56].

The positive value for remission formation and re-entry prevention of maintenance therapy combined with occupational therapy and occupational therapy is also emphasized (66).

It was found that 2-24 months after discharge from hospital exacerbations developed in 80% of patients who received placebo, in 80% of patients who received placebo and psychosocial therapy, in 53.9% of patients who received chlorpromazine, while when chlorpromazine was combined with psychosocial therapy - only in 37.3% of patients.

The follow-up study of patients with schizophrenia who had an acute relapse and were discharged to the family found less relapse and less prominence of deficit symptoms in the group of patients who were treated with an individually selected combination of neuroleptics combined with family psychotherapy than in the other group of patients who received the same therapy with neuroleptics combined with individually targeted psychotherapy.

The possibilities of biological and psychosocial interventions during remission in schizophrenic patients are confronted by the progredient tendencies of the biological process, about which our knowledge remains limited to certain limits.

Therefore, further resolution of this issue is closely related to the restoration or compensation of the defective biological systems and structures that play an essential role in the pathogenesis of the disease [164].

At the same time, the biological aspect of the problem of rehabilitation in schizophrenia is underdeveloped, which equally applies to one of the relevant modern areas of biological psychiatry - immunobiology.

Familiarization with few works carried out in this direction showed that schizophrenia patients reveal changes in different parts of immunological system not only during exacerbations and relapses of the disease, but also in remission periods.

It is also believed, judging by a number of investigated immunological indicators, that a stable and complete remission is achieved when psychobiological reactivity is normalized at all levels of neuropsychiatric activity [164]. When immunobiological reactivity determined by neuroautoimmune processes is insufficiently restored, remission in schizophrenia patients is usually unstable, despite seemingly stabilizing levels of improvement according to clinical observation. Thus, at present, the effectiveness of gradually and flexibly administered outpatient psychopharmacotherapy and environmental therapy is not in doubt.

At the same time, a review of the literature shows that, due to insufficient research on the role of various clinical, psychosocial, and immunological factors in the course of schizophrenic remissions, approaches to determining the prognosis of their course and choosing the optimal individual medical tactics are often empirical in nature.

The practical value of such multifactorial models of remission course in schizophrenia consists, first of all, in the fact that they would reflect certain complex prognostic criteria of clinical course of disease as well as would allow to define rational approaches to choice of an individual medical rehabilitation tactics including a complex of means and methods of both biological, including immunocorrective, and social influence on patients during remission.

The essence of this connection consists in the fact that in patients with schizophrenia with increase of duration of disease the sensitization of organism to cerebral antigens increases. This circumstance, in turn, has a negative influence on the course of remissions. We have already discussed the influence of other factors on remissions in this group of patients in the previous sections of this chapter.

This mathematically systematized complex of signs is not only clinical and pathogenetic, but also prognostic model of remission course, allowing taking into account clinical and immunological parameters established in patients to determine further clinical development of the disease. At the same time, based on the detected model of clinical and immunological manifestations of the course of remission, the use of desensitizing agents, aimed at eliminating and preventing further development of neuroallergic processes in the body of patients, seems pathogenetically justified.

Thus, the multifactorial model of clinical and immunological manifestations of the course of remission in patients with schizophrenia shows that prognosis of clinical development of the disease should be conducted taking into account a number of social (support in life, family relations, material and living conditions of the patient) and immunological factors of the results of determination of anti-brain incomplete antibodies and level of sensitization of organism to brain antigens.

Stabilization of remissions and prevention of relapses in this category of patients should be carried out by means of complex biosocial influence directed to strengthening of support in life and living conditions of the patient, elimination of psychosocial stresses, and also immunocorrective therapy including immunosuppressive and desensitizing agents.

CONCLUSION

There are conflicting data and disagreements among scientists about the various issues of prevalence, formogenesis, treatment efficacy, and course of remission in schizophrenia, mostly due to a one-sided clinical, biological, or sociological approach to the subject.

At certain stages of cognition such approaches were adequate and sufficient, but in the process of development of specific sciences it became evident the need to study also the regularities of the relationship of the processes under study, which allows to formulate a coherent theory of the development of the pathological process in mental illness.

A proper understanding of the role of various internal and external, biological and social factors in the etiopathogenesis and clinical course of schizophrenia is essential to overcome the seeming disjointedness of the earlier findings and to choose scientifically valid approaches to the theoretical and practical challenges facing psychiatry.

Therefore, the further development of schizophrenia doctrine and its progress is closely related to the scientific development of theory and means of methodology.

All this points to a significant increase in the role of modern scientific methodology, which should perform the task of synthesizing, integrating the obtained knowledge and ensure its further development at a higher level.

This corresponds to the principle of systems approach in scientific research, which involves the study of any object in the integrity of its integrative quality, in the fullness of its interrelated properties, in the unity of its internal and external relations.

The systems approach is understood as a method of cognition of objects that are complex systems to identify the mechanism of their vital functions, structure, laws of functioning and development.

As a human being is an open system with a very high degree of complexity, medicine, more than any other scientific discipline, is interested in a complex system approach to a human being, to the study of his health and illnesses.

The systemic approach to human pathology, i. e. 3e. the study of it as a system expresses an objective tendency to study its biosocial nature holistically.

Developing methodological issues of psychiatry, the leading psychiatric scientists also link the prospects for further study of the clinic and pathogenesis of mental disorders with a systematic approach to the subject of research and scientifically valid analysis of the findings.

Complex system approach to the study of the pathogenesis and course of mental illness from the position of correlation between social and biological allows us to avoid descriptiveness and one-sidedness of the research, to reveal general, linking into a single whole the mechanism of disease development, its internal regularities and their correlation with the surrounding social environment.

However, so far there are only isolated attempts to reveal this relationship in the light of a systemic approach to man.

The great clinical polymorphism of schizophrenia and the existing differences in its outcomes have attracted the attention of researchers since the establishment of the nosological independence of the disease.

Existing classifications of schizophrenia have been influenced by specific methodological approaches, as well as by changing philosophical, social, and general biological views of researchers. This has resulted in different classifications of the disease, as well as inconsistent results and a one-sided understanding of the role of heredity and the surrounding social environment in the formation and prognosis of schizophrenia.

At the same time, the differentiation of schizophrenia into basic forms of course, which show stability during the life of patients, already contains prognostic information and therefore the study of the role of social and biological in the form formation of the disease is continuously connected with its prognosis.

Defending the nosological unity of schizophrenia, we consider its occurrence and polymorphism of clinical forms as a result of interaction of hereditary and environmental factors.

The lack of sufficiently convincing correlations between the clinical forms of schizophrenia and the isolated effect of these factors prompts the need for a comprehensive approach to the questions of the extent to which the endogenous and exogenous, biological and social factors analyzed determine such significant clinical differences in the course of the disease.

It should be emphasized that none of the above factors had a specific influence on the formation and prognosis of the course of schizophrenia. On the contrary, certain complexes of nonspecific hereditary, clinical-biological, social and immunobiological factors corresponded to the clinical forms of schizophrenia, the integration of which determined the qualitative peculiarity of the form-forming mechanisms in schizophrenia.

A direct correlation was revealed in these groups between the severity of psychopathological disorders and the content of anti-brain autoantibodies in the blood.

The detected patterns confirm the feasibility of a comprehensive approach to the assessment and prediction of the course of schizophrenia.

Multifactorial models of relationships between clinical and biological, socio-psychological and immunological factors in various clinical forms of schizophrenia can be used for differential diagnosis and individual prognosis of the course of the disease as well as in the choice of rational means and methods of treatment of patients to reduce the progredient properties of the process.

Thus, the conducted systemic study of clinical and immunological relations in schizophrenia has shown that not an isolated factor, but features of interaction between different parts of the immune system in unity with other organism systems and the surrounding social environment, as well as the internal picture of the disease reflect the biosocial mechanism of disease development and specificity of its clinicopathological manifestations.

In the light of the findings, treatment efficacy and remission stability in schizophrenia are the result of an integral response of differentiated systems of clinical, immunological and socio-psychological factors whose composition and specific relationship features are determined by the clinical form of the disease course.

The established models of psychosocial and immunological relationships that reflect the mechanisms of disease development can be used in clinical practice for evaluation of individual prognosis of disease development, and also point to the necessity of system approach to the choice of rational therapeutic tactics that includes means of both biological, including immunocorrective, and psychocorrective influence on patients.

In schizophrenia as a multifactorial disease, a complex system of interaction between genetic, immunological and other biological factors with clinical, psychological and social factors determines the form and type of the disease course, prognosis and effectiveness of treatment with psychotropic agents, stability of remission, as well as ways to find correction of immunopathological processes.

The degree of disease progression is related to the intensity of the immunological response in the form of hypersensitivity to neurospecific proteins.

The quality of therapeutic remissions and their stability within different clinical forms of schizophrenia correlate not only with clinical as well as social factors, but also with the dynamics of immunological shifts.

The influence of clinical and socio-psychological factors on the effectiveness of therapy and the stability of remissions can be mediated by immunological processes. Unfavorable microsocial environment (conflictual relationships in the family, lack of social support, poor material and living conditions) as well as inadequate internal picture of the disease has a stressful effect on the immune system of the schizophrenia patient, contributing to sensitization of the body by brain antigens and activation of synthesis of immunoglobulins as well as anti-brain autoantibodies.

In various clinical forms of schizophrenia, the detection of incomplete anti-brain autoantibodies and hypersensitivity of peripheral leukocytes to brain antigens in the blood of patients expresses resistance to therapy and instability of remissions.

This substantiates the search for not only immunosuppressive, but also immunosuppressive therapy in different types of reactivity.

We were interested in the structure of the internal picture of the disease, i.e., the inner world of the patient through his eyes. And this representation on the psychological level coincides with the immunological state. It is possible to assume, that the change of one must entail the change of the other. This view opens up new possibilities and new ways of treating schizophrenia with immunological and psychocorrective methods.

What happens on the psychological level is mirrored in the body, in this case the immunological level.

The correspondence we found between the indicators of psychological and immunological statuses can be figuratively expressed in the form of the following parallels presented in Table 6.1.

Correlations between psychological and immune status indicators

Psychological status	Immunological status
1. the personality splits, and one part is not recognized as one's own, it is regarded as someone else's	1. The brain tissue's own proteins are not recognized and are considered by the organism as foreign
2. To someone else's part of the personality - fear, anxiety, aggression, desire to destroy	2. To the "foreign" protein - autoantibodies are produced, which are autoaggressive, destroying
3. due to the "alien" presence, the psyche is on "alert" or tense - the general level of anxiety increases	3. presence of antigens, besides autoantibodies, stimulates nonspecific immune system response - total amount of antibodies, immunoglobulins, lymphocytes increases.
4. Sensory automatism is present as part of Kandinsky-Clerambaud syndrome, the structure of which includes senestopathies, senestalgias.	4. Histamine is involved in a non-specific immune system response - its blood levels are elevated, it contributes to increased permeability of the GEB, and is also responsible for pain sensation
5. The patient is accessible to "alien influences, damaged ostensibly from outside, but actually by himself (the "wood and glass" symptom)	5. Nerve tissue becomes accessible, nerve cell membranes are damaged as the physicochemical properties of membrane and cytoskeletal proteins change and histamine contributes to increased permeability of the GEB.
6. Schizophrenic patients have very few somatic and infectious diseases, as they are under constant nervous tension.	6. High immunity prevents the development of somatic and infectious diseases.
7. A part of the personality becomes alien, posing a danger.	7. Part of the brain tissue is not recognized by its own immune system.
8. General personality anxiety is elevated.	8. Immunological composition of blood is strained - many changes.

The study of neurospecific proteins makes it possible to refine the diagnosis of schizophrenia, establish the duration of the disease and predict its progression. The data presented and the presence of autoantibodies to neurospecific antigens in the sera of patients with schizophrenia can be useful in the diagnosis of this disease.

In   addition, we developed a special scale for assessing the level of social adaptation of patients (Scheme 1), which along with clinical and psychological methods can use the technique of detecting autoantibodies to neurospecific antigens in the sera of patients. The scale synthesizes the data of clinical and psychopathological examination, the results of experimental and psychological examination, and the presence and level of neurospecific proteins in blood serum. Each item of the scale is expressed numerically. The sum of points is plotted on a straight line, the ends of which are the poles of complete adaptation and complete maladaptation, respectively. With the help of this technique it is possible to visually establish the level of social adaptation of the patient at present, his "problem areas", and to predict the future.

Social Adaptation Assessment Scale Figure 1

Qualities to be assessed	*Criteria and Scores*						
1. attitude towards oneself	inadequate -3	-2	-1	indifferent 0	+1	+2	adequate +3
2. attitude towards family	negative -3	-2		neutral 0			positive +3
3. attitude towards the past	negative -3			neutral 0			positive +3
4. attitude towards future	negative -3			neutral 0			positive +3
5. attitude towards others	negative -3			neutral 0			positive +3
6. anxiety	high -3			medium 0			low +3
7. aggressiveness	high -3			medium 0			absent +3
8. introversion-extroversion		pronounced introversion -3				pronounced extroversion +3	
9. psychoproduction	expressed -3			weak 0			absent +3
10. negative symptomatology	expressed -3			weak 0			absent +3
11. remission quality		0 -3	D -2	S -1	B 0		A +1
12. self-care	no -3			reduced 0			normal +3
13. work capacity	no -3			decreased 0			normal +3
14. criticism	no -3			reduced 0			normal +3
15. neurospecific proteins	expressed reaction -10			minimal 0			absent +10
Full Pole Full Pole							
maladaptation	-52			0			+52 adaptation

CONCLUSIONS

1. For the first time the complex method allowing to establish synchronous correlations between clinical, psychological and immunological condition of patients with schizophrenia and giving immunological substantiation of the phenomenon of "cleavage" in schizophrenia.

2. The appearance of the neurospecific protein N-CAM in the blood of schizophrenic patients, indicating cellular rearrangement, degeneration of cellular components and increased synaptogenesis, was found for the first time to be a marker verifying the presence of schizophrenic process in a psychiatric patient, provided there is no organic pathology.

3. For the first time reliable correlations between the intensity of neurospecific protein N-CAM formation in blood serum and the duration of the disease in patients with schizophrenia without an aggravating organic pathology in the anamnesis were revealed.

4. Consideration of the obtained data regarding synchronous changes in mental and immunological status of schizophrenic patients allows to modify treatment and rehabilitation measures, to combine therapy with psychotropic drugs with immunomodulators and psychocorrection more precisely and reasonably.

5. The developed criteria of investigation of clinical and immunological correlations in combination with the method of evaluation of the level of social adaptation of patients with schizophrenia, integrating the data of clinical and psychological and immunological examination, allow early detection, prevention of relapses and prognostication of schizophrenia in each specific case.

LIST OF REFERENCES

1. Avedisova A. S. Noncompliance or refusal of psychopharmacotherapy / A. S. Avedisova, V. I. Borodin // Ros. psikhiatr. zhurn. 2006. - – № 1. - – С. 61-65.

2. monoaminoxidase activity and indicators of endogenous intoxication in patients with first-episode schizophrenia / M. G. Uzbekov [et al. Neurology and Psychiatry. - – 2009. - – № 5. - – С. 24-27.

3. Actual problems of social and rehabilitation psychiatry in Ukraine / Tabachnikov S.I., Gorban Є. M., Mikhailov B.V. [and others] // Medical research. - – 2001. - Vol. 1, issue 1. - P. 6-8.

Alexandrovsky Y. A. Psychiatry and psychopharmacotherapy. - Moscow: GEOTAR-Media, 2004. - – 430 с.

5. Alfimova M. V. Our destiny - in our genes / M.V. Alfimova, V.E. Golimbet // Nature. - – 2003. - – № 6 – С. 13-18.

6. Apoptosis in schizophrenia: genetic and psychopharmacological factors / S. A. Ivanova [et al.] // Siberian Bulletin of Psychiatry and Narcology. - – 2005. - – № 37. - – С. 7-13.

7. Lymphocyte apoptosis in patients with paranoid schizophrenia / N.V. Ryazantseva [et al. - – 2007. - – № 9 – С. 56-56.

8. Berezovskaya M. A. Features of cerebral hemodynamics and microcirculation in patients with schizophrenia (review of literature) // Siberian Bulletin of Psychiatry and Narcology. - – 2011. - – № 67. - – С. 119-120.

9. Berezovskaya M. A. A. Results of study of cerebral hemodynamics in patients with paranoid schizophrenia // Zabaykalskii medic. vestnik. - – 2011. - – № 2. - – С. 23-28.

10. Berezovskaya M. A. A. Doppler assessment of cerebral blood flow in patients with paranoid schizophrenia / M.A. Berezovskaya, V.V. Kozlov // Siberian Medical Review. - – 2011. - – № 5. - – C. 20-23.

11. Wasserman L.I. Medical psychodiagnostics / L.I. Wasserman, O.Y. Shchelkova / In the book Theory, practice and training. - M.: Academia, 2004. - – 736 c.

12. Verbenko V. A. EEG reactivity in schizophrenia // Journal of Psychiatry and Medical Psychology. - – 2008. - – № 1. - – C. 30-35.

13. Voloshin P.. Voloshyn P. V., Maruta N. O. The strategy of psychiatric health protection of the population of Ukraine: modern possibilities and problems / P. V. Voloshyn, N. O. Maruta // Ukrainian Journal of Psychoneurology. - – 2015. - Vol. 23, vp. 1 (82) – C. 5 – 11.

14. Vorobyev V. M. On prevention and therapy of mental adaptation disorders / V. M. Vorobyov, N.L. Konovalova // Review of Medical Psychology and Psychiatry. V.M. Bekhterev. - – 1993. - – № 1. - – C. 71–72.

15. Vorobyev V. M. M. Mental adaptation as a problem of medical psychology and psychiatry / V.M. Vorobyev // Review of medical psychology and psychiatry named after Bekhterev. V.M. Bekhterev. - – 1993. - – № 2. - – C. 33–39.

16. Vostrikov V. M. Reduced numerical density of pericapillary oligodendrocytes in cerebral cortex in schizophrenia // Journal of neurology and psychiatry. - – 2007. - – № 12. - – C. 58-65.

17. High-tech approaches reveal conformational changes in the albumin molecule in patients with first-episode schizophrenia / M.G. Uzbekov [et al.] // Siberian Bulletin of Psychiatry and Narcology. - – 2013. - – № 76. - – C. 26-29.

18. Gamma rhythm, positive, negative symptoms and cognitive dysfunction in schizophrenia / V. B. Strelets [et al] // Journal of neurology and psychiatry. - – 2010. - – № 1. - – C. 77-83.

19. Glantz S. Medico-Biological Statistics / S. Glantz; translated from English by Yu. - M.: Practica, 1999. - – 459 c.

20. Govorin N. V. Peculiarities of disorders of lipid peroxidation processes in paranoid schizophrenia / N.V. Govorin, T.P. Zlova // Social and Clinical Psychiatry. - – 1999. - – № 4. - – C. 53-59.

21. Golimbet V. E. Serotonin and schizophrenia / V.E. Golimbet, M.V. Alfimova // Nature. - – 2012. - – № 8 – C. 34-38.

22. Gorobets L. N. Prolactin and peripheral sex hormone secretion in patients with first episode schizophrenia / L. N. Gorobets, M. I. Matrosova // Journal of neurology and psychiatry. - – 2010. - – № 10. - – C. 17-22.

23. Gubler E.V. Application of nonparametric statistical criteria in medical and biological research / E.V. Gubler, A.A. Genkin. - L.: Medicine, 1973. - – 142 c.

24. Denisov E. M. Metabolic disorders in patients with paranoid schizophrenia // Journal of Psychiatry and Medical Psychology. - – 2011. - – № 1. - – C. 24-30.

25. Dynamics of the contents of antibodies to neuroantigens in blood serum of patients with schizophrenia in the course of therapy / T.P. Klushnik [et al] // Journal of neurology and psychiatry. - – 2008. - – № 8. - – C. 61-64.

26. Differentiation of clinical variants of schizophrenia on the basis of parameters of electrodermal activity / S.A. Yagoda [et al.] // Medical Bulletin of North Caucasus. - – 2011. - – № 3. - – C. 105-106.

27. State of Health Report for Europe: Health and Health Systems, 2009. [Electronic resource]. - HERB VOS, 2010. Access mode : http://www.euro.who.int/PubRequest?language=Russian. - Screen title.

28. World Health Report. Mental Health: New Understanding, New Hope. - WHO, World Health Organization, 2001. - – 217 c. (WHO. The world health report 2001: MentalHealth: New Understanding, New Hope, 2001.)

29. Zhilyaeva T.V. Disorders of single-carbon metabolism in schizophrenia // Psychiatry and psychopharmacotherapy. - – 2012. - – № 6. - – C. 41-46.

30. Zhilyaeva T.V. Folate metabolism disorders in the light of dysontogenetic Hypotheses of schizophrenia etiology // Social and Clinical Psychiatry. - – 2012. - – C. 88-94.

31. Zaichenko A. A. A. Biometric indicators of constitutional risks of development of paranoid schizophrenia in men / A. A. Zaichenko, E. A. Lebedeva // Saratov Scientific-Medical Journal. - – 2009. - – № 3. - – C. 384-389.

32. Changes in the composition of erythrocyte membrane fatty acids in patients with first episode schizophrenia / N.V. Govorin [et al] // Siberian Bulletin of Psychiatry and Narcology. - – 2011. - – № 2. - – C. 9-12.

33. Changes in antibodies to nerve growth factor and interhemispheric asymmetry by level of constant brain potential in children from high risk group for schizophrenia / M.A. Kalinina [et al] // Asymmetry. - – 2010. - – № 3. - – C. 14-22.

34. Immune system in juvenile schizophrenia / G. I. Koliaskina [et al] // Siberian Bulletin of Psychiatry and Narcology. - – 2008. - – № 48. - – C. 22-26.

35. Karvasarsky B.D. Clinical psychology / B.D. Karvasarsky. - Peter, 2006. - – 959 c.

36. Clinical psychiatry: from a synopsis on psychiatry. In 2 vols. VOL. 1 / G.I. Kaplan, B.J. Sadok - Moscow : Medicine, 1994 - 672 p.

37. Clinical Psychiatry: translation from English supplemented / T.B. Dmitrieva [et al] - Moscow: "Medicine", 1998 - 528 p.

38. Klushnik T.P. Immune system and schizophrenia: clinical and biological interrelations (review of the state of the problem) / T.P. Klushnik, I.V. Scherbakova // Psychiatry. - – 2005. - – № 6. - – C. 48-61.

39. Klyushnik T.P., Lebedeva I.S., Shcherbakova I.V., Orlova V.A., Lideman R.R. Interrelation of neurophysiological and immunological markers of active current schizophrenic process // Journal of neurology and psychiatry. S. S. Korsakov. - – 2005. - – T.105, №10. - – C. 42-46.

40. Kozlovskaya G.V., Klushnik TP, Kalinina MA, Shcherbakova IV, Golubeva N.I. Preliminary results of a new immunomodulator Roncoleukin in the complex therapy of children with schizophrenia // Journal of Psychiatry and Psychopharmacotherapy. P.B. Gannushkin. - – 2005. - – T.7, №5. - – C.259-262.

41. Kolesnichenko E. V. Features of lipid peroxidation and neurotrophic regulation in schizophrenia // Saratov scientific medical journal. - – 2008. - – № 3. - – C. 81-83.

42. To the problem of neurodegeneration in schizophrenia: data of spectral dynamic analysis / V.A. Orlova [et al] // Social and Clinical Psychiatry. - – 2010. - – № 2. - – C. 67-78.

43. Kolomeyets N. S. Intercellular interactions in human brain in schizophrenia (ultrastructural-morphometric study): abstract of Ph. ... Cand. of Biological Sciences : 03.03.04 / Natalya Stepanovna Kolomeets. - Moscow, 2010. - – 49 c.

44. Kolomeyets N.S. Changes of synaptic contacts on dopaminergic neurons of black substance in schizophrenia (immunocytochemical study) / N.S. Kolomeyets, N.A. Uranova // Materials of All-Russian conference "Interaction of experts in rendering assistance at mental disorders", October 27-30, 2009. - – 2009. - – C. 382.

45. Kolomeets N.S. The significance of microglia reactivity in brain pathology in schizophrenia // Journal of Neurology and Psychiatry. - – 2009. - – № 109. - – C. 60-63.

46. Complex neurochemical estimation of brain proteins in norm and at schizophrenia / G.Sh. Burbaeva [et al] // Journal of neurology and psychiatry. - – 2008. - – № 2. - – С. 44-50.

47. Kondratenko M. Y. An analysis of theories of etiology and pathogenesis of schizophrenia / M. Y. Kondratenko // Actual issues of modern medicine and pharmacy : proceedings of an additional scientific-practical conference with international participation of young scientists and students, 13-17 of January 2019. - Zaporizhia: ZDMU, 2019. - – С. 66-67.

48. Criterion for quality of life in psychiatric practice / N.A. Maruta, T.V. Panko, I.A. Yavdak, [et al]. - X.: REEF ARSIS, LTD, 2004. - – 239 с.

49. Iznak A. F. Disorders of structural and functional organization of the brain in schizophrenia // Psychiatry. - – 2008. - – № 3. - – С. 25-31.

50. Study of some indicators of oxidative stress in blood adolescents in schizophrenia and mental retardation / E. B. Burlakova [et al] // Psychiatry. - – 2009. - – № 3. - – С. 15-21.

51. Lagun I. Я. Causality of schizophrenia / I.Y. Lagun. - Lipetsk: OAO "PK Orius", 2008. - – 289 с.

52. Lapach S. N. N. Statistical methods in medical and biological research using Excel / S. N. Lapach, A. V. Chubenko, P. N. Babich. - K.: Morion, 2000. - – 320 с.

53. Lytayev S.A. Fundamentals of clinical psychology and medical psychodiagnostics / S.A. Lytayev, B.V. Ovchinnikov, I.F. Diakonov. - 2nd ed. - Saint-Petersburg: ELBI-SPb. 2008. - – 316 с.

54. Langle A. Psychopathology and existential themes in schizophrenia // Moscow Psychotherapeutic Journal. - – 2008. - – № 4. - – С. 37-57.

55. Magnetic resonance imaging of frontal lobes in schizophrenia: correlation with serum levels of antibodies to nerve growth factor / I. V. Shcherbakova [et al] // Journal of neurology and psychiatry. - – 2009. - – № 3. - – С. 44-46.

56. Mazaeva N. A. Schizophrenia: prenatal and postnatal risk factors // Journal of Neurology and Psychiatry. - – 2012. - – № 5. - – C. 98-107.

57. Markers of endothelial dysfunction in preexisting-progressive schizophrenia // I. V. Scherbakova [et al] // Journal of Neurology and Psychiatry. - – 2005. - – № 3. - – C. 43-46.

58. Maruta N. A. Restoration of social functioning is the main goal of depression therapy / N. A. Maruta // Neuronews. - – 2013. - – № 8 (53). - – C. 16-20.

59. Matrosova M. I. The role of sex hormones in pathophysiology of the first episode of schizophrenia / M. I. Matrosova, Gorobets L.N. // Social and Clinical Psychiatry. - – 2011. - – № 4. - – C. 31-33.

60. Medical psychology: state national manual / I.D. Spirina, I.S. Vitenko, O.K. Naprenenko [and others]. - Dnipropetrovsk : PE "Lira" Ltd. 2012. - – 444c.

61. International Classification of Diseases (10th revision). Classification of clinical and mental disorders. Clinical descriptions and guidelines for diagnosis. - K. : Fact, 1999. - – 272 c.

62. Möller H.-J. Schizophrenia: Current concepts and therapeutic consequences // Psychiatry and Psychopharmacotherapy. - – 2011. - – № 3. - – C. 8-13.

63. Multiparametric combinatorial analysis of EEG rhythms in norm and in schizophrenia / V. B. Strelets [et al. I. P. Pavlov. - – 2007. - – № 6. - – C. 684-691.

64. Ministry of Health of Ukraine. Order N 59 of 5.02.2007 'On the Approval of Clinical Protocols for Medical Care in the Psychiatric Specialty'. - K.: Chancellor's Office, 2007. - – 44 c.

65. Mosolov S. N. N. Scales of psychometric assessment of schizophrenia symptomatology and the concept of positive and negative disorders / S.N. Mosolov. - – M., 2001. - – C. 96-144.

66. MRI-parameters of subcortical and frontal brain structures as markers of schizophrenia susceptibility / N.N. Efanova [et al] // Russian Psychiatric Journal. - – 2005. - – № 5. - – C. 12-15.

67. Napreko O. K. State of psychiatric care in Ukraine in 2003 and the last decade, ways of its improvement / O. K. Naprenko, V. V. Dobrovolska // Journal of Psychiatr. and Medical Psychology. - – 2004. - – № 3 (13). - – C. 3-7.

68. Napreyenko O. K. K. Psychiatric science in Ukraine in 2013 and tensions of its improvement (according to the data of the Problem Commission "Psychiatry" of the MOH and NAMS of Ukraine) / O.K. Napreyenko // Ukrainian Newsletter of Psychoneurology. - – 2014. -Vip. 1 (78) – C. 18-22.

69. Naumov A. V. The role of methylation processes in etiology and pathogenesis of schizophrenia / A. V. Naumov, Yu. E. Razvodovsky // Journal of neurology and psychiatry. - – 2009. - – № 8. - – C. 91-98.

70. Existence disorder in schizophrenia / E. Yu. Zavershneva [et al] // Moscow Psychotherapeutic Journal. - – 2005. - – № 2. - – C. 65-90.

71. Disruption of conformation of serum albumin binding centers in schizophrenia / E. Yu. Michionzhnik [et al] // Journal of neurology and psychiatry. - – 2008. - – № 5. - – C. 67-70.

72. Disturbance of glutamate metabolism at schizophrenia / G.Sh. Burbaeva [et al] // Bulletin of Russian Academy of Medical Sciences. - – 2007. - – № 3. - – C. 19-23.

73. Disturbance of production and receptor of tumor necrosis factor alpha in patients with paranoid schizophrenia / A.P. Melnikov [et al] // Bulletin of Siberian Branch of RAMS. - – 2007. - – № 6. - – C. 37-43.

74. Some immune and metabolic aspects of schizophrenia pathogenesis / V. M. Frolov [et al] // Russian psychiatric journal. - – 2006. - – № 6. - – C. 33-37.

75. Regulatory framework of clinical trials of psychotropic drugs in Ukraine / O. Naprenenko, V. Usenko, I. Spirina. [and others] // Newsletter of pharmacology and pharmacy. - – 2006. - – № 12. - – C. 19-26.

76. Obyedkov V. G. New data on the nature of genetic polymorphism and their importance for theoretical models of schizophrenia // Medical Journal. - – 2004. - – № 1. - – C. 18-23.

77. Orlov V. A. Regularities of free-radical processes in schizophrenia // Fundamental'nye issledovanie. - – 2012. - – № 8. - – C. 215-219.

78. Peculiarities of the immune system state in endogenous mental diseases with marked affective disorders / S.A. Zozulya [et al.] // Journal of Neurology and Psychiatry. - – 2011. - – № 12. - – C. 63-67.

79. Peculiarities of fatty acid composition of erythrocyte membranes in patients with the first psychotic episode of schizophrenia / A. S. Ozornin [et al] // Zabaikal Medical Bulletin. - – 2011. - – № 1. - – C. 79-83.

80. Features of spectral power of EEG rhythms in children with early childhood autism and their relationship to the development of various symptoms of schizophrenia / E. A. Lushchekina [et al] // Journal of Higher Nervous Activity. I. P. Pavlov. - – 2011. - – № 5. - – C. 545-552.

81. Pathology of oligodendroglia and myelinated fibers in the hippocampus in schizophrenia (ultrastructural-morphometric study) / N.S. Kolomeyets [et al] // Journal of Neurology and Psychiatry. - – 2008. - – № 108. - – C. 52-60.

82. Search for biomarkers and development of pharmacogenetic approaches to personalized therapy of patients with schizophrenia / S. A. Ivanova [et al.] // Siberian Bulletin of Psychiatry and Narcology. - – 2013. - – № 76. - – C. 12-17.

83. Polymorphisms of interleukin-1 (IL-1B) and interleukin receptor antagonist (IL-1RN) genes in schizophrenia / V. E. Golimbet [et al. Neurology and Psychiatry. - – 2012. - – № 12. - – C. 63-68.

84. Prenatal stress as a risk factor for schizophrenia and bipolar affective disorder / G.I. Brekhman [et al.

Ivanovo Medical Academy. - – 2010. - – № 1. - – C. 23-29.

85. Psychiatry and drug treatment: a handbook / O.K. Naprenenko [and others]. - Kyiv: VSV "Medicine", 2011. - – 528 c.

86. Psychiatric Clinic: a tutorial for students and interns / Ed. by V. P. Samokhvalov. P. Samokhvalov. - Simferopol, 2003. - – 608 c.

87. Psychology of corporeality: theoretical and practical research: collection of articles from the 2nd international scientific-practical conference / Ed. by E. V. Burenkov. - Penza: PGPU named after V.G. Belinsky, 2009. - – C. 148-157.

88. Putyatin G. G. Putyatin / In book: Abramov V. A. Psychosocial rehabilitation of patients with schizophrenia / V. A. Abramov, I. V. Zhigulina, T. L. Ryapolova. - Donetsk: Kashtan, 2009. - – C. 65 – 110.

89. Rachkauskas G.S. Dynamics of functional and morphological indices of microhemocirculation in patients with paranoid schizophrenia with therapeutic resistance when using polioxidonium and alpha-tocopherol / G.S. Rachkauskas, V.M. Frolov, I.I. Kutko, M.O. Peresadin // Ukrainian morphologic almanac. - – 2009. - – T. 7, № 2. - – C. 87-91.

90. Rebrova O. Statistical analysis of medical data. Application of applied software package STATISTICA / Rebrova O. Yu. - Moscow : Media Sphere, 2002. - – 312 c.

91. Correlation between parameters of platelet serotonin system and clinical signs of psychosis at patients with attack-progressive schizophrenia / Brusov O.S. [et al] // Journal of neurology and psychiatry. - – 2007. - – № 7. - – C. 17-24.

92. Skripnikov A.M., Kidon P.V. Etiology and pathogenesis of schizophrenia: Present-day state of study of the problem. - Poltava: ASMI, 2019. - – 51 c.

93. Senkov O. Dark Matter of the Brain: Schizophrenia // In the World of Science. - – 2010. - – № 5. - – C. 29-38.

94. Modern look at the basic pathogenetic hypotheses of schizophrenia / T.P. Klushnik [et al] // Psychiatry. - – 2010. - – № 1. - – C. 7-13.

95. Sonnyk G.T. Psychiatry / G.T. Sonnyk, O.K. Naprenenko, A.M. Skripnikov. - Kyiv: "Zdorov'ya", 2006. - – 432 c.

96. State of innate and acquired immunity in children from high risk group of schizophrenia and children with schizophrenia / T.P. Klushnik [et al] // Journal of neurology and psychiatry. - – 2005. - – № 11. - – C. 45-49.

97. Spectral power and intracortical interactions by beta2-rhythm in norm and schizophrenia / V. B. Strelets [et al. I. P. Pavlov. –2004. - – № 2. - – C. 229-236.

98. State of the Mental Health of the Population and Mental Health Care in Ukraine: Informational and Analytical Review 2000-2009. M.P. Zhdanova, M.V. Golubchikov, P.V. Voloshyn [and others] / Ministry of Health of Ukraine and others. - Kharkiv : Arsis, 2010. - – C. 8–16.

99. State of mental health of the population and prospects for the development of psychiatric care in Ukraine [Text] / Khobzei M.K., Voloshin V. V., Maruta N. O. and others. // Ukrainian Journal of Psychoneurology. - – 2012. - T. 20, vol. 3(72). - – C. 13-18.

100. Structural features of a brain at patients with schizophrenia and their relatives on the data of the morphometric analysis of MRI-images of a brain / E.A. Miloserdov [et al] // Social and clinical psychiatry. - – 2005. - – № 15 (1). - – C. 5-12.

101. Uzbekov M. G. The first episode of schizophrenia is accompanied by changes in activity of blood aminoxidases // Neurochemistry. - – 2009. - – № 4. - – C. 337-340.

102. Pharmacotherapy in neurology and psychiatry / ed. by S.D. Enna, J.T. Coyle; transl. from English - Moscow : Medical Information Agency, 2007. - – 800 c.

103. Characteristics of EEG alpha rhythm during the first episode of paranoid schizophrenia / Melnikova T. S. [et al] // Social and Clinical Psychiatry. - – 2013. - – № 1. - – C. 40-45.

104. Khobzey M.K. Socially-oriented psychiatric support in Ukraine: Problems and solutions / M.K. Khobzey, P.V. Voloshyn, N.O. Maruta // Ukrainian Newsletter of Psychoneurology. - – 2010. - T. 18, vol. 3 (64). - – C. 10-14.

105. Khoyetsyan A. G. G. The role of abnormalities of brain development in pathogenesis of schizophrenia / A. G. Khoyetsyan, A. S. Boyajyan // Journal of Neurology and Psychiatry. - – 2010. - – № 2. - – C. 97-101.

106. Frequency and character of metabolic disorders in patients with schizophrenia / N.G. Neznanov [et al] // Review of Psychiatry and Medical Psychology. - – 2009. - – № 2. - – C. 17-20.

107. Schizophrenia as a progressive disease of the brain / N. E. van Haren [et al] // Social and Clinical Psychiatry. - – 2008. - – № 2.– C. 26-35.

108. Shmukler A. B. Structural and functional discordance of different parts of brain in schizophrenia: role of introgressive perception // Social and Clinical Psychiatry. - – 2010. - – № 3. - – C. 86-95.

109. Shcherbakova I. V. Activation of innate immunity in schizophrenia // Journal of neurology and psychiatry. - – 2006. - – № 10. - – C. 79-82.

110. Shcherbakova I.V., Klushnik T.P. Immune system and schizophrenia: clinical and biological interrelations (review of the state of the problem) // Psychiatry (Scientific and Practical Journal). - – 2005. - – №6 (18). - – C. 48-62.

111. Shcherbakova IV, Siryachenko TM, Sarmanova ZV, Kaleda VG, Barkhatova AN, Lideman RR, Klushnik TP Some indicators of the state of

innate and acquired immunity in patients with endogenous schizophrenic spectrum diseases // Journal of neurology and psychiatry. S.S. Korsakov. - – 2005. - – T.105, №3. - – C.47-51.

112. Shcherbakova I.V., Klushnik T.P., Kozlovskaya G.V., Kalinina M.A. State of innate and acquired immunity in children at high risk of schizophrenia and children with schizophrenia. //Journal of neurology and psychiatry. S.S. Korsakov. - – 2005. - – T.105, №11. - – C. 45-9.

113. Yagoda S.A. Biomarkers of schizophrenia and ways of objectivization of psychopharmacotherapy // Modern therapy of psychiatric disorders. - – 2011. - – № 2. - – C. 2-7.

114. Yanshin P. V. Practicum on clinical psychology. To be able to use these techniques in order to develop a personality / P. V. Yanshin. - SPb., 2004. - – 336 c.

115. Yastrebov V. S. Self-stigmatization of patients with major psychiatric diseases / V. S. Yastrebov, I. I. Mikhaylova // Journal of Neurology and Psychiatry. C. C. Korsakov. - – 2005. - – № 105 (11) – C. 50-54.

116. Abel T. Epigenetic targets of HDAC inhibition in neurodegenerative and psychiatric disorders / T. Abel, R. S. Zukin // Current opinion in pharmacology. - – 2008. - – № 8. - – P. 57-64.

117. Abnormal anterior cingulum in patients with schizophrenia / Z. Sun [et al.] // Neuroreport. - – 2003. - – № 14. - – P. 1833-1836.

118. A new approach to remediating problem-solving deficits in outpatients with moderate-to-severe cognitive impairments / D. Langenbahn, J. Rath, A. Hradil [et al.] // Arch. Phys. Med. Rehab. - – 2008. - Vol. 89. - Abstracts of an American Congress of Rehabilitation Medicine, October 15-19, 2008, Toronto, ON, Canada. - – E11.

119. Anterior cingulum abnormalities in male patients with schizophrenia determined through diffusion tensor imaging / F. Wang [et al] // American Journal of Psychiatry. - – 2004. - – № 161. - – P. 573-575.

120. Apoptosis and schizophrenia: A pilot study based on dermal fibroblast cell lines / V.S. Catts [et al.] // Schizophrenia research. - – 2006. - – № 84. - – P. 20-28.

121. Apoptotic mechanisms and the synaptic pathology of schizophrenia / L. A. Glantz [et al.] // Schizophrenia research. - – 2006. - – № 81. - – P. 47-63.

122. Apoptotic mechanisms in the pathophysiology of schizophrenia / L. F. Jarskog [et al] // Progress in neuropsychopharmacology & biological psychiatry. - – 2005. - – № 29. P. 846-858.

123. Association between the BBNF gene and schizophrenia / P. Muglia [et al.] // Molecular psychiatry. - – 2003. - – № 8. - – P. 146-147.

124. A systematic review and meta-analysis of Northern Hemisphere seasons of birth studies in schizophrenia / G. Davies [et al] // Schizophrenia Bulletin. - – 2003. - – № 3. - – P. 587–593.

125. Benezech M. Mental patients and death at Cadillac psychiatric hospital: A 30-year study (1923-1952) // Annales Medico-Psychologiques. - – 2011. - – V. 169(1). - – P. 63-69.

126. Bleakley S. Identifying and reducing the risk of antipsychotic drug interactions // Progress in Neurology and Psychiatry. - – 2012. - – V. 16(2). - – P. 20-24.

127. Bolonna A. A. Partial agonism and schizophrenia / A. A. Bolonna, Kerwin R. W. // Therapeutics of Mental Disorders. - – 2006. - – № 2. - – C. 31-34.

128. Brown A. S. Prenatal infection as a risk factor for schizophrenia // Schizophrenia Bulletin. - – 2006. - – № 2. - – P. 200–202.

129. Carlsson A. The neurochemical circuitry of schizophrenia // Pharmacopsychiatry. - – 2006. - – № 39. - – P. 10-14.

130. Chronic schizophrenia as a brain misconnection syndrome: a white matter voxelbased morphometry study / G. Spalletta [et al.] // Schizophrenia research. - – 2003. - – № 1. - – P. 15-23.

131. Cingulate fasciculus integrity disruption in schizophrenia: a magnetic resonance diffusion tensor imaging study / M. Kubicki [et al.] // Biological psychiatry. - – 2003. - – № 54. - – P. 1171-1180.

132. Clarke M. Evidence for an interaction between familial liability and prenatal exposure to infection in the causation of schizophrenia // Schizophrenia research. - – 2008. - – № 102. - – P. 41-48.

133. Contribution of methylenetetrahydrofolate reductase (MTHFR) polymorphisms to negative symptoms in schizophrenia / J. L. Roffman [et al] // Biological psychiatry. - – 2008. - – № 63. - – P. 42-48.

134. Davies Eric J. Developmental aspects of schizophrenia and related disorders: possible implications for treatment strategies // Advances in psychiatric treatment. - – 2007. - – № 13. - – P. 384-391.

135. Epigenetic therapeutic strategies for the treatment of neuropsychiatric disorders: ready for prime time? / S. I. Deutsch [et al.] // Clinical neuropharmacology. - – 2008. - – № 2. - – P. 104-119.

136. Fact sheet #104 [electronic resource] / World Health Organization. - Geneva: WHO, 2015. - Retrieved from: http://www.who.int/mediacentre/factsheets/fs104/en/. - published 01.10.15.

137. Focal white matter density changes in schizophrenia: reduced inter-hemispheric connectivity / H. E. Hulshoff Pol [et al.] // Neuroimage. - – 2004. - – № 1. - – P. 27-35.

138. Joint Formulary Committee. British National Formulary. - London: BMJ Group and Pharmaceutical Press, 2014. - – 1144 p.

139. Global, regional, and national age-sex-specific all-cause and cause-specific mortality for 240 causes of death, 1990-2013: A systematic analysis for the Global Burden of Disease Study 2013 / M. Naghavi, H. Wang, R. Lozano [et al.] // The Lancet. - – 2015. - – V. 385(9963). - - – 117-171.

140. Gottesman I. I. The endophenotype concept in psychiatry: etymology and strategic intentions / I. I. Gottesman, T. D. Gould, and others, American Journal of Psychiatry, 2003. - – № 160. - – P. 636-645.

141. Grabe H. J. Alexithymia and personality in relation to dimensions of psychopathology / H. J. Grabe, C. Spitzer, H. J. Freyberger // Amer. J. Psychiatry. - – 2004. - Vol. 161. - – P.1299–1301.

142. Gray Matter Volume Decreases in Elderly Patients with Schizophrenia: A Voxel-based Morphometry Study / C. Schuster [et al.] // Schizophrenia bulletin. - – 2011. - – № 37. - – № 1.

143. Harrison P. J. Schizophrenia genes, gene expression, and neuropathology: on the matter of their convergence / P. J. Harrison, D. R. Weinberger, L. et al. 2005, Molecular psychiatry. - – № 10. - – P. 40-68.

144. High glycine levels are associated with prepulse inhibition deficits in chronic schizophrenia patients / U. Heresco-Levy [et al] // Schizophrenia research. - – 2007. - – № 91. - – P. 1-3, 14-21.

145. Hickie I. B. Are common childhood or adolescent infections risk factors for schizophrenia and other psychotic disorders? / I. B. Hicke, R. Banati, C. H. Stewart, A. R. Lloyd. - – 2009. - – V. 190(4). - – P. 17-21.

146. Homocysteine, methylenetetrahydrofolate reductase and risk of schizophrenia: a metaanalysis. / J.W.. Muntjewerff [et al.] // Molecular psychiatry. - – 2006. - – № 11. - – P. 143-149.

147. Impaired flush response to niacin skin patch among schizophrenia patients and their nonpsychotic relatives: the effect of genetic loading / S. S. Chang [et al.] // Schizophrenia bulletin. - – 2009. - – № 1. - – P. 213–221.

148. Incipient neurovulnerability and neuroprotection in early psychosis / G. E. Berger [et al.] // Psychopharmacology bulletin. - – 2003.– № 37. - – P. 101.

149. Instability of prefrontal signal processing in schizophrenia / G. Winterer [et al] // The American Journal of psychiatry. - – 2006. - – № 11. - – P. 1960-1968.

150. Ito C. The role of the central histaminergic system on schizophrenia // Drag news perspective. - – 2004. - – № 17. - – P. 383-387.

151. Javitt D.C. Glutamate and Schizophrenia: Phencyclidine, N-Methyl-d-Aspartate Receptors, and Dopamine-Glutamate Interactions // International Review of Neurobiology. - – 2007. - – № 78. - – P. 69-108.

152. Kim T. H. Serum homocysteine and folate levels in Korean schizophrenic patients // T. H. Kim, S. W. Moon // Psychiatric investigation. - – 2011. - – № 8. - – P. 134-140.

153. Konrad A. Disturbed structural connectivity in schizophrenia - primary factor in pathology or epiphenomenon? Konrad, G. Winterer // Schizophrenia Bulletin. - – 2008. - – № 1. - – P. 77-92.

154. Mayilan K. R. The complement system in schizophrenia / K. R. Mayilan, D. R. Weinberger, R. B. Sim. // Drug news & perspectives. - – 2008. - – № 4. - – P. 200-210.

155. Metabolic changes in schizophrenia and human brain evolution / P. Khaitovich [et al.] // Genome biology. - – 2008. - – № 9. - – P. 124.

156. Miller C. L. The Evolution of Schizophrenia: A Model for Selection by Infection, with a Focus on NAD // Current Pharmaceutical Design. - – 2009. - – V. 15. - – P. 100-109.

157. Molecular genetics of schizophrenia: a critical review / N. Berry [et al.] // Journal of psychiatry and neuroscience. - – 2003. - – № 28. - – P. 415-429.

158. Morphometric analysis of lateral ventricles in schizophrenia and healthy controls regarding genetic and disease-specific factors / M. Styner [et al] // Proceedings of the National Academy of Sciences of the United States of America. - – 2005. - – № 102 (13). - – P. 4872-4877.

159. Mortality in schizophrenia and related psychosis: data from two cohorts, 1875-1924 and 1994-2010 [electronic publication] / D. Healy, J. Le Noury, M. Harris, M. Butt [et al.] // BMJ Open. - – 2012. - V.2 - e001810. - retrieved from: http://bmjopen.bmj.com.

160. MRI assessment of gray and white matter distribution in Brodmann's area of the cortex in patients with schizophrenia with good and poor outcomes / S. A. Mitelman [et al] // American journal of psychiatry. - – 2003. - – № 12. - – P. 2154-2168.

161. MRI study of white matter diffusion anisotropy in schizophrenia / B. A. Ardecani [et al.] // Neuroreport. - – 2003. - – № 16. - – P. 2025-2029.

162. Naber D. A self-rating to measure subjective effects of neuroleptic drugs, relationships to objective psychopathology, quality of life, compliance and other clinical variables / D. Naber // Int Clin Psychopharmacol. - – 1995. - vol. 10. - Suppl. 31. – P. 133 – 138.

163. Neural cell adhesion molecule-associated polysialic acid regulates synaptic
plasticity and learning by restraining the signaling through GluN2B-containing NMDA receptors / G. Kochlamazashvili [et al.] // Journal of neuroscience. - – 2010. - – № 30 (11). - – P. 4171-4183.

164. Neuroanatomical abnormalities before and after onset of psychosis: a cross-sectional and longitudinal MRI comparison / C. Pantelis [et al.] // Lancet. - – 2003. - – № 361. - – P. 281-288.

165. Neurobiology of early psychosis / M.S. Keshavan [et al] // British journal of psychiatry. - – 2005. - – № 187. - – P. 8-18.

166. Neuregulin 1 transcripts are differentially expressed in schizophrenia and regulated by 5' SNPs associated with the disease / A. J. Law [et al] // Proceedings of the National Academy of Sciences. - – 2006. - – № 103. - – P. 6747-6752.

167. Neuroplasticity and schizophrenia / D.O. Frost [et al.] // Biological psychiatry. - – 2004. - – № 56. - – P. 540-543.

168. Overproduction of neutrophil radical oxygen species correlates with negative symptoms in schizophrenic patients: parallel studies on neutrophil

chemotaxis, superoxide production and bacterial activity / P. Sirota [et al.] - – 2003. - – № 2. - – P. 123-132.

169. Pathways that make voices: white matter changes in auditory hallucinations / D. Hubl [et al] // Archives of general psychiatry. - – 2004. - – № 7. - – P. 658-668.

170. Picker J.D. Do maternal folate and homocysteine levels play a role in neurodevelopmental processes that increase risk for schizophrenia? D. Picker, J. T. Coyle // Harvard review of psychiatry. - – 2005. № 13. - – P. 197-205.

171. Plasma homocysteine, folate and B12 in chronic schizophrenia / A. Haidemenos [et al] // Progress in neuro-psychopharmacology & biological psychiatry. - – 2007. - – № 31. - – P. 1289-1296.

172. Polischuk I. I. Effect of various extrinsic factors on the course of schizophrenia // Zhurnal Nevrologii i Psikhiatrii imeni S. S. Korsakova. - – 1982. - – V. 82(5). - – P. 98-102.

173. Poor premorbid adjustment and CT scan abnormalities in chronic schizophrenia / D.R. Weinberger [et al] // American journal of psychiatry. - – 1980. - – № 137. - – P. 1410-1413.

174. Prenatal exposure to influenza as a risk factor for adult schizophrenia / F. Limosin [et al] // Acta Psychiatrica Scandinavica. - – 2003. - – № 5. - – P. 331–335.

175. Production of proinflammatory cytokines correlates with the symptoms of acute sickness behavior in humans // U. Vollmer-Conna [et al.] // Psychology medical. - – 2004. - – № 7. - – P. 1289-1297.

176. Progressive structural brain abnormalities and their relationship to clinical
outcome: a longitudinal magnetic resonance imaging study early in schizophrenia / B. C. Ho [et al] // Archives of general psychiatry. - – 2003. - – № 60 (6). - – P. 585-594.

177. Rates of adult schizophrenia following prenatal exposure to the Chinese famine of 1959-1961 / D. St Clair [et al.] // Journal of the American Medical Association. - – 2005. - – № 294. - – P. 557-562.

178. Reelin and glutamic acid decarboxylase67 promoter remodeling in an epigenetic methionine-induced mouse model of schizophrenia / E. Dong [et al.] // The Proceedings of the National Academy of Sciences of the United States of America. - – 2005. - – № 102. - – P. 12578—12583.

179. S-adenosyl methionine and DNA methyltransferase-1 mRNA overexpression in psychosis / A. Guidotti [et al.] // NeuroReport. - – 2007. - – №18. - – P. 57-60.

180. Schizophrenia risk from complex variation of complement component 4 / A. Sekar [et al.] // Nature. - – 2016. - – № 530. - – P. 177-183.

181. Schizophrenia: Medical illness, mortality, and aging / D. A. Casey, M. Rodriguez, C. Northcott [et al.] // International Journal of Psychiatry in Medicine. - – 2011. - – V. 41(3). - – P. 245-251.

182. Shoval G. The possible role of neurothrophins in the patogenesis and therapy of schizophrenia / G. Shoval, A. Weizman // European neuropsychopharmacology. –2005. - – № 3. - – P. 319-329.

183. Sharma T. Cognition in schizophrenia. Impairments, importance, and treatment strategies / T. Sharma, Ph. Harvey // University Press, Oxford. 2000. - – 263 p.

184. Structural neiroimaging in adolescents with a first psychotic episode / D. Moreno [et al] // Journal of the American Academy of child and adolescent psychiatry. - – 2005. - – № 44 (11). - – P. 1151-1157.

185. Structural disconnectivity in schizophrenia: a diffusion tensor magnetic resonance imaging study / J. Burns [et al] // British journal of psychiatry. - – 2003. - – № 182. - – P. 439-443.

186. Subtle disruption of the middle cerebellar peduncles in patients with schizophrenia / G. Okugawa [et al.] // Neuropsychobilogy. - – 2004. - – № 50. - – P. 119-123.

187. The application of DTI to investigate white matter abnormalities in schizophrenia / M. Kubicki [et al] // Annals of New York Academy of sciences. - – 2005. - – № 1064. - – P. 134-148.

188. The immune system and schizophrenia: an integrative view / N. Muller [et al.] // Annals of New York Academy of sciences. - – 2000. - – № 917. - – P. 456-467.

189. Wang J. Perceived Effectiveness of Mental Health Care Provided by Primary-Care Physicians and Mental Health Specialists / J. Wang, S. B. Patten // Psychosomatics. - – 2007. - Vol. 48. - – P. 123-127.

190. White matter volume changes in people who develop psychosis / M. Walterfang [et al.] // International journal of neuropharmacology. - – 2004. - – № 7. - P. S258-S259.

191. The kynurenic acid hypothesis of schizophrenia / Erhardt S. [et al.] // Physiology and behavior. - – 2007. - – № 10. - – P. 203-209.

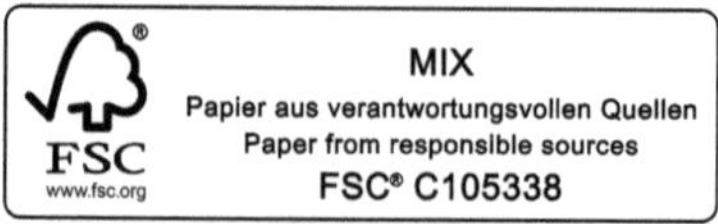

Printed by Books on Demand GmbH, Norderstedt / Germany